Adoption

and

Ethics

A SERIES BY MADELYN FREUNDLICH

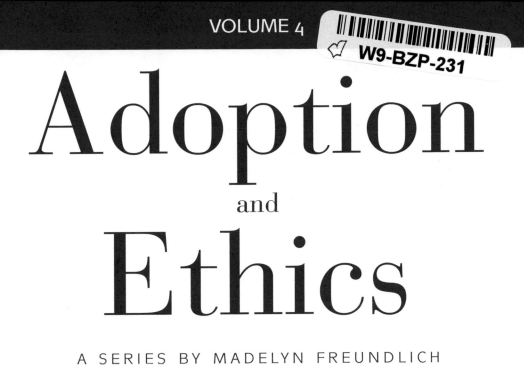

ADOPTION AND ASSISTED

REPRODUCTION

CHILD WELFARE LEAGUE OF AMERICA

THE EVAN B. DONALDSON ADOPTION INSTITUTE

CWLA Press is an imprint of the Child Welfare League of America. The Child Welfare League of America is the nation's oldest and largest membership-based child welfare organization. We are committed to engaging people everywhere in promoting the well-being of children, youth, and their families, and protecting every child from harm.

CHILD WELFARE LEAGUE OF AMERICA, INC.
HEADQUARTERS
440 First Street, NW, Third Floor, Washington, DC 20001-2085
E-mail: books@cwla.org

CURRENT PRINTING (last digit)
10 9 8 7 6 5 4 3 2 1

Cover design by James D. Melvin
Text design by Peggy Porter Tierney

Printed in the United States of America

ISBN # 0-87868-807-2

Library of Congress Cataloging-in-Publication Data
Freundlich, Madelyn.
    Adoption and assisted reproduction/ by Madelyn Freundlich.
       p. cm.
    Includes bibliographical references.
    ISBN 0-87868-807-2
    1. Adoption--United States. 2. Reproductive technology--United
States. 3. Adoption--Moral and ethical aspects. 4. Reproductive
technology--Moral and ethical aspects.   I. Child Welfare League of
America. II. Title.
    HV875.55 .F728 2001
    362.73'4'0973--dc21

                                                          2001017489

Contents

Preface

This title is the fourth in a series of publications developed by the Evan B. Donaldson Adoption Institute and published by the Child Welfare League of America. The series is part of the Adoption Institute's multiyear initiative focused on ethical issues in adoption. It is designed to provide the field with a synthesis of the current base of knowledge on key adoption policy and practice issues—issues that currently pose challenges to adoption professionals and that are likely to confront the field in the future. This volume on adoption and assisted reproduction follows earlier publications on the role of race, culture, and national origin in adoption; market forces in adoption; and the impact of adoption on members of the triad.

Why a Focus on Ethics in Adoption

Adoption is a complex subject, with social, psychological, legal, and cultural dimensions. It is shaped by policy—at the international, national, state, county, and agency levels—and by practice—on the part of social workers, attorneys, judges, mental health professionals, and others. It involves the needs, interests, and rights of children, birth parents, relatives, foster parents, adoptive parents, and adult adoptees. Adoption includes domestic adoptions of healthy newborns, international adoptions of children from dozens of countries with widely varying policies, and adoptions of children in foster care in this country. Because of this complexity, adoption has been and continues to be the subject of much debate. The controversies in adoption have extended across a spectrum of policy and practice issues, and although the contentious issues have become clear, resolution has not been achieved nor has consensus developed regarding a framework on which to further quality adoption policy and practice.

Productive outcomes have been hindered by the constituency-based considerations that have shaped, to a great extent, the tenor of the debate. Emotion and rhetoric have come to characterize much of the discussion and, as a result, it has been difficult to focus on substantive issues in a reasoned and informed manner or clarify the goals and principles that can assist in resolving the many points of disagreement. From the divisive debates on access to identifying information, to the emotionally-laden controversies on transracial adoption, to the increasingly intense disputes over the competing "rights" of members of the adoption triad—the environment surrounding adoption has become highly charged and focused efforts to craft quality policy and practice more difficult to achieve.

The Adoption Institute, in collaboration with leading thinkers in the field of adoption from across the country, approached this environment by proposing an ethics-based framework for analyzing and resolving the complex challenges in adoption. The decision to utilize an ethics-based approach was based, first, on a belief that ethics could provide a method for reframing the critical issues in adoption and avoiding the divisiveness that has impeded the resolution of the key challenges. Second, the choice of an ethics-based approach was based on an assessment that such a framework would support the identification of the range of issues that impact contemporary adoption, the analysis of relevant considerations from multiple perspectives, and the development of a course of action for improving future policy and practice. The Adoption Institute's ethics initiative has three major components:

- an identification and examination of the core values and principles that underlie quality adoption policy and practice;

- thorough analyses of the critical policy and practice issues that demand attention; and

- the development of a strategy that draws on a sound knowledge base to advance quality adoption policy and practice in the future.

The Critical Issues in Adoption

Because adoption is complex, bringing to the fore many competing interests, values, perspectives, and constituencies, it is not an easy task to reach consensus on which issues represent the most critical questions. The Adoption Institute approached this challenging process by first bringing together a multidisciplinary Ethics Advisory Committee. The members of this group represent a rich diversity of professional backgrounds and expertise, including adoption practice and policy, clinical psychology, sociology, political science, the law, the judiciary, bioethics, medicine, medical anthropology, religion, and social science research. With the guidance of this Committee, the Adoption Institute identified key ethical issues that affect adoption policy and practice and prioritized the most critical issues for in-depth analysis and action. The following topics were selected as critical areas for ongoing attention and work:

Adoption and Assisted Reproduction

This topic, the focus of this volume, raises the question of whether assisted reproduction (including sperm donation, egg donation, and embryo transfer), which may result in a child who is not genetically related to one or both parents, creates a situation that is analogous to adoption. Should the knowledge that has been acquired in the field of adoption be applied in the area of assisted reproduction? Are issues in adoption—such as identity, access to background information, and search—equally applicable in the context of reproductive technology? Should any or all adoption practice standards apply?

The Role of Race, Culture, and National Origin in Adoption

This topic—on which a previous volume focused—considers critical questions regarding the role of race, culture, and national origin in adoption from the perspective of individuals served by adoption and from a broad policy perspective. In this complex area of adoption policy and practice, there are many unresolved questions related to the role of race, culture and national origin in an adoptee's personal identity and the extent to which racial and cultural similarities and differences between adoptive parents and children should be taken into account. These questions have been placed at the forefront of the policy debate as a result of recent changes in federal law, which now prohibits consideration of race in the adoptive placement of children in foster care; debates related to the Indian Child Welfare Act; and the mandates of the Hague Convention on Intercountry Adoption.

The Market Forces in Adoption

This topic—also the focus of a previous volume—considers various aspects of the "business" of adoption in terms of market factors. With the shifting demographics of infant adoption, international adoption, and special needs adoption, issues are raised about the role of money in adoption, who holds the "power" in adoption, and to whom adoption professionals are accountable. Increasingly, the field of adoption struggles with such questions as: To what extent has there been a commodification of children who are placed with adoptive families? How is the adoption process regulated and by whom? How are the roles of birth and adoptive parents affected by differences in resources? Is the concept of accountability relevant to adoption, and if so, how? Do market forces undermine ethical adoption practice?

The Impact of Adoption on Adopted Persons, Birth Parents, Adoptive Parents, and Adoptive Families

This topic—the focus of a previous volume—focuses on the many ways that adoption may impact each member of the adoption triad. For the adopted person, adoption may affect the individual's overall adjustment and well-being, as well as the ability to develop a personal identity. What are the outcomes for adopted persons and to what extent do past and current adoption practices affect those outcomes? For the birth parent, adoption practice and law may impact, both in the short and long term, an individual's sense of personal integrity. To what extent are birth parents well-served by adoption and how do societal perceptions of birth parents affect their sense of well- being? For adoptive parents, adoption involves achieving parenthood in a nontraditional way. To what extent does being "approved" to parent impact adoptive parents? Do adoptive families face special challenges in a society that accords primacy to biological bonds?

The Ethics in Adoption Series

Essential to knowledgeable discussion and issue resolution in each of these four areas is a sound understanding of the current knowledge base—the research, the practice-based knowledge, and the policy analyses advanced by leading thinkers in the many fields bearing on adoption: social work, law, psychology, child and adolescent development, medicine, and education. The four publications that form the series are designed to provide a synthesis of the existing knowledge base that can inform and challenge thinking and analysis in each of the critical topic areas. They outline the key issues; review the current data, including statistical information to the extent it exists; identify the research that addresses the key issues; describe the current practice-based knowledge; and synthesize the policy arguments that have been advanced and debated. Whenever possible, the strengths and weaknesses of various perspectives are assessed.

The publications, including this volume on adoption and assisted reproduction, are not designed to take a position on the issues or advance a specific viewpoint as to what is "ethical" or "unethical." It is only through ongoing discussion that consensus can be reached as to what represents the most ethical course of action in adoption—for those directly touched by adoption and for those who provide professional adoption services. It is hoped that the publication series will provide a tool for furthering this discussion—a springboard for advancing adoption policy and practice currently and into the future.

Introduction

With recent developments in assisted reproduction providing greater opportunities to create nongenetic parent-child relationships, the interface between assisted reproduction and adoption has become more apparent. Sperm donation has been an established procedure for more than a century and has long played a role in assisted reproduction.[1] In vitro fertilization (IVF)—using the egg and sperm of the intended parents—has become an increasingly recognized infertility treatment since the 1978 birth of Louise Brown, the first child conceived with this reproductive technology.[2] More recent approaches derived from IVF technology, that is, egg donation[3] and embryo donation,[4] result in children with no genetic connections with one or both of their intended parents. These emerging assisted reproduction services suggest closer analogies to adoption than previously was the case, and they raise important issues about the extent to which adoption and assisted reproduction are similar or distinctly different ways of non-traditional family formation.

Assisted reproduction, like adoption, has moved into public awareness and achieved some level of social acceptance. Assisted reproduction has, in fact, outpaced adoption in some respects. In the United States each year, approximately 60,000 births result from donor insemination, 15,000 births result from in vitro fertilization, and about 1,000 births result from surrogacy [Institute for Science, Law and Technology 1998]. By comparison, between 25,000 and 30,000 infants are adopted each year in the United States [Carstens 1995]. The interface between assisted reproduction and adoption has not been extensively studied. Increasingly, however, adoption language is being used to refer to certain reproductive technologies. It is not altogether uncommon to find the adoption of existing children referred to as "traditional adoption" as distinguished from the practice of embryo donation, which is characterized as "embryo adoption" [see Embryo Adoption 1999]. Some writers have begun to refer to assisted reproduction services using donated gametes in adoption language as well. Holbrook [1990, p. 334], for example, writes that artificial insemination may involve, in some respects, the "adoption of a sperm," and notes that the practice of egg donation and surrogacy may be viewed as taking "a diametrically opposed approach that might be characterized as the adoption of an egg via 'rental' of a womb." Are embryos and eggs "adopted" by their recipients? Is assisted reproduction with donor gametes a variant of adoption? What do references to assisted reproduction in adoption language suggest about adoption?

From one perspective, the two methods of family formation are quite distinct. The environments in which each service is provided are different; the extent to which medical, psychosocial, and legal circumstances are predominant vary; and the longer-term implications of each service may differ. On the other hand, adoption and assisted reproduction have much in common. Both, to a great extent, originate with infertility, and each serves not as a cure for infertility but as an alternative means to build a family. Neither assisted reproduction nor adoption is typically an individual's first choice in terms of building a family. In both forms of family formation, there are likely to be implications of the choice for all parties concerned over the entire life cycle. It is also clear that both adoption and assisted reproduction challenge the traditional view of family as based on genetic or biological ties and raise questions about personal identity and the environments in which families are formed in nontraditional ways [Benward 1999].

There are many complex issues that arise in adoption and assisted reproduction involving the use of donated sperm, eggs, and embryos, and an in-depth discussion of these issues is beyond the scope of this volume. The general parameters of some of these issues, however, will be addressed: adoption and assisted reproduction as alternatives for infertile individuals; the achievement of parenthood through each of the two means of nontraditional family formation; the issues confronting the parties served through adoption and assisted reproduction; the role of anonymity in adoption and assisted reproduction; the extent to which market forces shape each service; the special considerations related to embryo donation; and the legal structures governing each service. Although the discussion generally will reference assisted reproduction, particular emphasis will be placed on those services that result in a child who is not genetically related to one or both of the intended parents as these services more closely parallel adoption.

Endnotes

1. Although artificial insemination of both humans and animals had been practiced in Europe since the early part of the 19th century, the first recorded insemination using the sperm of a donor took place in the United States in 1884 [Blyth 1999].

2. In vitro fertilization (IVF) is "the union of sperm and egg in a laboratory dish, literally 'in glass' rather than inside the body" [New York State Task Force on Life and the Law 1998, p. 52]. The intended mother is given ovarian stimulating drugs; the egg is removed, fertilized with sperm in the laboratory, and implanted into the mother's uterus. The intended father's sperm is usually used, although it is possible to use sperm donation in conjunction with IVF [New York State Task Force on Life and the Law 1998]. In 1996, a total of 20,659 babies were born as a result of the 64,036 ART cycles carried out that year using one of the following procedures: IVF (involving the extraction of a woman's eggs, fertilization of the eggs in the laboratory, and then the transfer of the resulting embryo(s) into the woman's uterus through the cervix); GIFT (gamete intrafallopian transfer) (used in 5% of procedures and involving the use of an instrument to help place the unfertilized eggs and sperm into the woman's fallopian tubes); and ZIFT (zygote intrafallopian transfer), (used in 2% of procedures and involving the fertilization of a woman's eggs in the laboratory and the transfer of the fertilized eggs (zygotes) into her fallopian tubes) [U.S. Department of Health and Human Services 1996].

3. In egg (or oocyte) donation, eggs are removed from a donor, fertilized in vitro and implanted in the intended mother, and, as a result, she is not genetically linked to the child. Although the intended father is often genetically linked to the child because his sperm is used, less commonly, the donated egg may be fertilized by donated sperm—in which case, neither intended parent is a genetic parent of the child. Pre-existing embryos conceived with a donor's egg also may be

implanted into a surrogate who becomes the gestational mother. This type of surrogacy (so-called gestational or carrier surrogacy)—in which the woman carries a fetus who has no genetic relationship to her—differs from traditional surrogacy in which the surrogate contributes her own egg for insemination with sperm from the male partner of the infertile couple [Seibel et al. 1993].

4. Embryo donation involves the implantation into an intended mother of a pre-existing frozen embryo created from another individual's IVF attempts and donated anonymously by these individuals [Embryo Adoption 1999]. In such cases, the resulting child is not genetically linked to the intended parents. As in egg donation, the intended mother may be the gestational mother or a surrogate may be enlisted to serve this role.

Chapter 1

Infertility, Assisted Reproduction, and Adoption

Conception, pregnancy, and child bearing are matters of ingrained importance in American culture. Historically, parenthood has been socially and culturally defined as deriving largely from biological relationships; there are expectations that a "flesh and blood" connection will exist between parent and child; adults are assumed to have the power to decide when they will become parents; bonding and attachment are viewed as the natural result of pregnancy and the birth process; and children are expected to physically and temperamentally resemble their parents to a greater or lesser degree [Daly 1992]. Shapiro [1982, p. 333] notes that individuals "grow up thinking that conception and giving birth are matters of choice"; consequently, when they experience infertility, it is generally "an unanticipated crisis" to which they react with shock and disbelief. Infertility may be a "major negative life event" with significant deleterious effects on the well-being of the individual [Abbey et al. 1992, p. 413] and adverse effects on the quality of married life [Ward 1998]. Infertility has been associated at the personal level with a diminished sense of self-esteem [Wright et al. 1991] and loss of a sense of internal control [Paulson et al. 1988]. At the interpersonal or couple level, infertility has been found to involve the loss of a common dream [Burns 1987]; a sense of threat to the infertile partner who knows that the other partner could have a child [Humphrey 1986]; anger because childlessness has been forced upon the couple [Butler & Koraleski 1990]; and a loss of sexual self-esteem in the context of the relationship [Shapiro 1993].

When confronted with infertility, many individuals seek assisted reproduction services in order to have a genetically related child, and in many cases, continue what may be costly,

1

painful and unsuccessful attempts to achieve that goal [Anderson 1989; Black et al. 1992; Goodman & Rothman 1984; Williams 1992]. Both the drive to find solutions to infertility and the tenacity with which individuals pursue assisted reproduction services raise questions regarding the existence of a "biological imperative." Are humans, as Winter writes [1997, p. 5], "driven by a primordial edict to bear children?" Some studies suggest that there may be an inherent psychological or social need to procreate. Bringhenti and associates [1997, p. 431], for example, found that "most women with infertility problems consider this condition to be a constant source of stress and one patient in two may even regard it as the most upsetting experience in her life." In a study of 61 men whose partners were unable to conceive and had sought alternative methods to have children, the researchers found that 40% of the men viewed a baby as the "essential completion of the family," 33% viewed having a baby as "the aim of life," and 16% said that a baby represented "the continuation of one's own self" [Chelo et al. 1986, p. 214].

Although it is clear that increasing numbers of individuals have sought medical treatment for infertility over the past 25 years [Stephen & Chandra 2000], relatively few infertile individuals seek to adopt. Winter [1997], for example, estimates that only about 11% of infertile adults pursue adoption. This low level of interest in adoption among infertile individuals suggests that assisted reproduction and adoption—if viewed as "competing"— may not be equally valued by those who seek a solution to infertility. Is reproductive technology the "winner"? Has adoption devolved from the second choice (behind traditional biological procreation) to the "third best" or even "fourth best" option, considered as a possibility only after assisted reproduction through in vitro fertilization and services using donor gametes have proven unsuccessful?

The literature strongly suggests that when prospective parents compare assisted reproduction and adoption, assisted reproduction easily achieves preferred status. Berg [1995, p. 81] writes of the powerful drive to have a biologically-related child:

> It is undeniable that among the individuals choosing to
> rear children, most prefer to have a biological child.
> Adoption is usually considered only when a (hetero-
> sexual) couple is unable to have a biological child. This
> nearly universal preference...reveals not only a value
> placed on the genetic linkage but on other aspects of the
> experience of parenting a biological child (e.g., the expe-
> rience of pregnancy and childbirth).

As a result, despite the high level of medically-related intrusion
and other physical and psychological demands, these technologies "afford the best approximation to the natural processes of
conception, gestation, and childbirth available to the infertile"
[Berg 1995, p. 84]. The New York State Task Force on Life and the
Law in its report, Assisted Reproductive Technologies: Analysis
and Recommendations for Public Policy [1998, p. 87], notes that
although the benefits of adoption are clear, "adoption does not
satisfy a desire to experience pregnancy or to raise one's genetic
offspring." Pointing to research that demonstrates limited interest
in adoption among infertile individuals, the Task Force noted that
many view adoption as "riskier than biological parenting and
lacking in certain valued experiences" [1998, p. 87]. "Riskiness"
is associated with the possibility that an adopted child will have
developmental, physical, or psychological problems because of
genetic or prenatal factors; the child will have a difficult time
coping with the fact that she is adopted; and the child's birth
parents may try to reclaim her at a later date [New York State Task
Force on Life and the Law 1998]. The "valued experiences" found
to be lacking in adoption are the experience of pregnancy and
childbirth and the continuation of the family line [New York State
Task Force on Life and the Law 1998]. Others assert that adoptive
and biological parenting are "equally valuable experiences" but
emphasize that the two means of parenting have many differences
and "some individuals may be better suited to one than to the
other" [Berg 1995, p. 84].

It is important to note that although the number of infertile
individuals who choose to adopt is low, the percentage of indi-

viduals who adopt because of infertility is high. Winter [1997], for example, estimates that about one-half of individuals who adopt newborns seek assisted reproduction services first. Berry, Barth, and Needell [1996] found in their research that high percentages of adopters had attempted to become pregnant before adopting. Their study revealed that 83% of those who adopted through private agencies, 80% of those who adopted independently, and 50% of those who adopted through public agencies had unsuccessful attempts at pregnancy. A large majority (86% of private agency adopters, 80% of independent adopters, and 49% of public agency adopters) reported that they adopted because they were unable to have a biological child. These findings tend to support a view of adoption as at most a "second best" alternative.

In assessing the relative benefits of assisted reproduction and adoption, infertile individuals are likely to opt in favor of assisted reproduction when it offers the opportunity to have a genetically related child and/or the gestational experience. When, however, the genetic linkage between intended parent and child is not a possibility, does assisted reproduction continue to hold preferred status? When there is no opportunity for a genetic linkage (as in the case of using both donated sperm and eggs), or a gestational experience (as in the case of surrogacy), or either (as in the case of embryo donation combined with surrogacy), does assisted reproduction continue to afford benefits that make it clearly preferable to adoption? The answers to these questions are not clear. The tensions related to the genetic, gestational, and social aspects of parenthood that these questions suggest, however, have implications for a range of issues that surface in adoption and assisted reproduction.

Chapter 2

The Meaning of Parenthood in Assisted Reproduction and Adoption

Adoption and assisted reproduction expand the concepts of "parent" and "family" from their traditional definition [Kirk 1985; Miall 1987; Williams 1992]. Adoption extends the concept of "parent" to individuals who socially and legally achieve that status after demonstrating the desire, capability, and intention to be fully responsible for raising the child. Assisted reproduction likewise expands the concepts of "parent" and "family," but in very different ways than does adoption. Unlike the sociolegal process of adoption that creates a nongenetic parent-child relationship, assisted conception offers intended parents the possibility of a biological and/or genetic parent-child relationship. In both adoption and assisted reproduction, however, there are tensions regarding parenthood. At one level, there are issues related to becoming a parent through nontraditional means, with psychological and social implications for individuals whose method of family formation is at odds with social and cultural expectations regarding becoming a "normal" family. At another level, there are issues related to the fact that multiple adults are involved in the process of family formation in both adoption and assisted reproduction. This reality can give rise to disputes among the parties as to who is the "real" parent of the child or offspring.

Becoming a Parent through Adoption or Assisted Reproduction

Because infertility underlies both adoption and assisted reproduction, it can be expected that individuals who achieve parenthood through either means share certain psychological experiences. The clinical literature and research, for example, suggest that the experience of infertility can impact subsequent parenting, particularly when individuals become parents through assisted reproduction [see Burns 1990] or through adoption [see Brodzinsky 1987; Humphrey & Humphrey 1988]. The achievement of parenthood through the two means may differ, however, in important ways.

Adoptive Parenthood

The clinical literature suggests that the decision to adopt often involves a difficult and uncertain transition from infertility to parenthood [Rosenberg 1992]. Individuals must confront the reality that biogenetic parenthood may not be possible and begin to view parenthood in social and interpersonal rather than biological terms [Rosenberg 1992]. The cultural emphasis on biological family formation as the "normal" way to become parents presents a series of psychological hurdles [Daly 1992; Hoffman-Riem 1990]. At the same time, in order to seriously consider adopting a child, infertile individuals must grieve the loss of the biologically related child that they always wanted but never had [Winter 1997].

Sandelowski [1995] describes the experiential course of infertile couples who, having made the decision to adopt, move toward the point at which a child will be placed with them. She finds that this time period involves certain unique psychological processes that distinguish the achievement of social parenthood from that of biological parenthood. First, she notes that adopters strive to "create a temporal order" in order to cope with the unmarked adoption waiting period [1995, p. 129]. Because the waiting time to adopt contrasts markedly with the fairly well-defined period of pregnancy, adopters often attempt to gain control over the uncertainty and avoid "living only to wait for a child" [1995, p. 129]. Second, she describes a process through which many adopters "construct or reconstruct a family romance" for the child. These family romances tend to take the form of a biography for the child that meshes with the adopters' own biography and emphasizes that the child is "loved" by them [1995, p. 129]. Finally, adopters tend to "stake a claim" in order to "own" the child as their own [1995, p. 130]. This "claiming" process principally involves adopters' concerns about themselves as "genuine" parents: anxieties about being "accepted" as the child's "real parents;" efforts to de-emphasize "the importance of the blood tie between parent and child;" and struggles to establish a "right" to their child "by emphasizing the close biological or biographical match between them and their child" [1995, p. 130]. Sandelowski observes that many adopters, as a result of these concerns, feel "fully parental" only after they have a child for a longer period of time than the birth parents or foster parents parented the child or after the adoption has been legally finalized [1995, p. 127].

Achieving Parenthood through Assisted Reproduction and Analogues to Adoption

Many of the psychological dynamics that characterize the achievement of adoptive parenthood may also be associated with achieving parenthood through assisted reproduction. In language that may aptly reflect the experiences of prospective adoptive parents, Braverman [1999, p. 8] notes that:

> The psychological adjustment to becoming parents through gamete donation is probably evolutionary—just like adjustments to other life changes. Parenting in general is thought to involve different stages, and the ability to parent effectively also changes with experience.

Just as the decision to adopt may carry with it psychological stresses associated with infertility, the decision to become parents through the use of donor gametes also may present significant stress for infertile adults. The decision is likely to take place at the same time that the couple is experiencing the cumulative effects of ongoing infertility treatment, attempting to understand complex medical information, and coping with the reality that one or both will not make a genetic contribution to the child [Braverman 1999]. Similarly, as may be the case when prospective adoptive parents are "matched" with a prospective birth mother whose infant is due within several months, gamete recipients may have feelings of excitement once a donor "match" is found "but also may experience feelings of fear, anxiety or loss" [Braverman 1999, p. 7]. Once the intended parents become aware that a donor has been identified, "the hypothetical donor is now real and, like all real people, has good as well as bad qualities. Old or new thoughts about what the child may look or act like or a reawakening of mourning the genetic connection may be stimulated by the donor match" [Braverman 1999, p. 7]. Likewise, there may be heightened anxiety after the child's birth. Braverman [1999, p. 8] notes that parents may feel concerned about the baby's physical characteristics that differ from those of the parents and may "express a deep concern that they may not be able to love or attach to the child because of the lack of a genetic bond."

The desire for physical similarity between parent and child is not unknown in adoption. Adoption, by its very nature, involves a nongenetic parent-child relationship created socially rather than biologically, but prospective adoptive parents may have certain expectations related to physical resemblance, which at minimum often involve an expectation of racial similarity [see Bartholet 1998]. Adoption practice of the 1950s and 1960s supported close physical similarities between the adoptive parent and child and espoused careful matching of prospective adoptive parents and children on physical and ethnic characteristics as well as other matters such as religion and social background. Such matching was undertaken to create an adoptive family that was as close to the biological family model as possible, thus preserving the secret that the family had adopted [Gill in press]. Beginning in the 1970s, efforts at close physical matching of parents and child began to decline as social work practice embraced a model of adoptive family formation that was clearly distinct from biological family formation [Kirk 1964].

Currently, the goals of physical similarity and "masking" adoptive families have all but disappeared. Adoption has become socially acceptable and adoptive families, consequently, no longer require shielding from public scrutiny. The pool of healthy infants in the U.S. has significantly diminished so that prospective adoptive parents (who are largely Caucasian), who greatly outnumber the Caucasian infants available for adoption, are now broadly accepting of children of diverse physical and ethnic characteristics. Further, the number of multicultural families in the U.S. has grown as a result of a number of factors, including increased rates of racial intermarriage and the growing number of international adoptions [Freundlich 2000]. These realities, however, raise questions about the attractiveness of adoption for adults who wish to have children who closely resemble them physically. Does assisted reproduction present a more appealing alternative for some individuals because they have the opportunity to select donors who "match" them physically and, consequently, they can "pass" as a "normal" biogenetic family (as adoptive families did previously)?

As in adoption, there are issues in assisted reproduction related to the impact of the absence of a genetic bond on parents' love for and attachment to their children. These pervasive concerns may arise from several sources, including, as Jean Benward [personal communication, June 26, 2000] notes, beliefs about the meaning of family, social stigma, and underlying anxieties about the "normalcy" of any family formed in ways other than voluntary intercourse between married partners [see Mahowald 1996]. These dynamics give rise to beliefs that the absence of a genetic tie may negatively impact the psychological status of children conceived through gamete donation because the quality of the parent-child relationship will be adversely affected and the child's sense of identity will be compromised as a result of less than full acceptance as a family member [Burns 1987, 1990].

The limited research in this area suggests that contrary to such expectations, there may be equal or, in some cases, greater parental involvement among donor recipient parents than parents who are genetically related to their children [Golombok et al. 1995; Golombok & Murray 1999]. In their study of different groups of parents, including parents who conceived by sperm donation, Golombok and associates [1995] found no differences in parent-child relationships between families in which sperm donation was utilized and parents with genetically related children who had utilized in vitro fertilization or parents who had adopted their children. The researchers concluded that the strong desire for parenthood might be far more powerful than genetic connections in promoting healthy parent-child relationships. In a subsequent study involving families in which the children were conceived following egg donation, Golombok and Murray [1999] found that the absence of a genetic connection between the mothers and children had no impact on the quality of the mothers' parenting, but, in fact, was associated with greater psychological well-being. The researchers [1999, p. 525] concluded:

> Infertile couples who choose to raise a child who is genetically unrelated to the mother may be even more committed to parenthood, and consequently find parenting a more satisfying experience than those who become mothers and fathers through other routes.

These findings contrast with findings of some clinical studies of adopted children that suggest that, among other factors [see Brodzinsky et al. 1998], the absence of a genetic relationship between a child and one or both parents may be associated with parent-child alienation and a higher level of psychological problems among children [Brodzinsky et al. 1995]. As Brodzinsky [1990] notes, however, outcomes for children are associated with multiple factors, including the age at which children enter families. The younger the child at time of adoption, for example, the less likely she is to exhibit emotional or behavioral problems [Brodzinsky 1990]. Taking these studies into account, Golombok and Murray [1999, p. 525] conclude that their findings of positive parenting outcomes in families created through gamete donation may apply to both "children raised from birth by a nongenetic parent" and "from early infancy in the case of adopted children." They [1999, pp. 525] state that these findings suggest that "the absence of a genetic relationship, in itself, does not lead to difficulties for parents or children."

The researchers also speculate that the discrepancy between their findings and the adoption literature may be explained on other grounds:

> It may be relevant that children born through egg or
> sperm donation do not experience the loss of an existing
> parent. Nor do they need to form relationships with new
> family members [Golombok & Murray 1999, p. 525-526].

The majority of the families studied by Golombok and Murray,
however, had not disclosed the donor conception status to their
children, and as a result, the children did not have knowledge of
a "genetic other" to whom they were related. Questions remain
regarding whether children conceived through gamete donation
and who know of their origins will perceive the donor as an
"existing parent" and experience a sense of loss in this regard.
Questions regarding offspring perceptions of donors as "parents"
in any meaningful sense of the term will be answered only through
studies of cohorts of donor offspring who have had full knowledge
of their donor conception status from childhood. Questions related to such offspring knowledge have important implications for
practice in the area of information disclosure and will be discussed later in more depth.

Disputes Regarding Who Is the "Parent"

Both adoption and assisted reproduction raise the question of the
essence of parenting. Is parenthood essentially genetic, gestational, or intentional without any necessary genetic or gestational
component? In adoption, is the "real" parent the birth parent or the
adoptive parent? In assisted reproduction, who among the individuals involved in bringing a child into being (potentially an egg
donor, a sperm donor, a surrogate, an intended mother, and an
intended father) is "the parent"? In both adoption and assisted
reproduction, these issues have played out most dramatically in
highly contentious court cases.

The "Parent" in Adoption

Because adoption is both a legal and social process, "parent" has a
relatively clear legal definition. Legally, adoption vests the adoptive
parents with all parental rights. As Macklin [1991, p. 6] notes:

In the case of adoption, a person or couple genetically unrelated to a child is deemed that child's legal parent or parents. The biological parent or parents of the child never cease to be genetically unrelated...but by virtue of law, custom, and usually emotional ties, the adoptive parents become the child's family.

That said, adoption disputes develop, albeit infrequently, among adults who each claim the child as theirs. Typically, courts are asked to resolve the competing claims of the birth mother or, in some cases, the birth father and the prospective adoptive parents. The asserted rights of birth mothers and birth fathers often are articulated in "genetic" or "biological" terms, and the asserted rights of the prospective adoptive parents often are stated in relation to their "psychological" or "social" parenting status. Courts have resolved these disputes based on legal—as opposed to ethical—considerations, although many have found these legal resolutions to be not altogether satisfactory [see Bartholet 1993; Hollinger 1995].

Constitutional principles as well as state statutes and case law play significant roles in defining the rights of birth parents in the context of adoption and the extent to which their interests in their children are recognized. The legal rights of birth parents have been expressly recognized by the United States Supreme Court, including the right to "marry, establish a home, and bring up children" [*Meyer v. Nebraska* 1923, p. 399]; the right to educate their children [*Wisconsin v. Yoder* 1972]; and the right to make reproductive decisions [*Griswold v. Connecticut* 1965]. Birth mothers' constitutional rights have been clearly defined and protected, reflecting the unique physical and social relationship between a mother and her child [*Planned Parenthood v. Casey* 1992; *M.L.B. v. S.L.J.* 1996]. Women, as a consequence, have recognized constitutional rights to make decisions regarding their pregnancies and regarding their children, including the right to make an adoption plan if they so choose [Craig 1998].

The rights of biological fathers are less clear. In 1983, the Supreme Court held that the "mere existence of a biological link" is not sufficient to bestow full constitutional protections on a birth father [*Lehr v. Robinson* 1983, p. 261]. When a birth father is married to the birth mother or is the legal father of a child (as in the case of the husband of the birth mother), he receives the same due process and equal protection constitutional rights as the biological mother [Craig 1998]. When a birth father, however, is not married to the birth mother and has not established himself legally as the father of the child, he has only an "opportunity interest," that is, a less-than-absolute right to the possibility of a parental relationship with his child [Craig 1998]. Although states are required to protect an unmarried father's interest in establishing such a parental relationship, they are free to define the specific conduct in which an unmarried father must engage in order to demonstrate that he has indeed assumed a parental role in his child's life [Craig 1998].

Courts often have ruled in favor of birth fathers in cases in which the men were denied the opportunity to plan for their children [see *In re Adoption of Doe* 1994]. In one case, for example, the court held that there was only one remedy for the lower courts' failure to vindicate "the real father": to take the baby from the "strangers" who had kept him "without right" and turn him over to the man who had a "preemptive right" to his child "without regard to the so-called best interests of the child" [*In re Adoption of Doe* 1994, p. 195]. Just as decisions in the leading assisted reproduction cases have been subject to debate, the decisions in contested adoption cases have been hotly disputed, with questions raised about whose interests should be recognized as most compelling.

Much of the debate in the adoption arena has centered on the applicability of the concept of "best interests of the child"—a concept that has no real analogue in assisted reproduction (an issue discussed later). Craig [1998, p. 413], on the one hand, argues against a "best interests of the child" standard. She maintains that "best interests of the child" is wholly subjective and, in particular, deprives unwed fathers of an opportunity interest before they even have the chance to pursue a relationship with their children. Hollinger [1995], on the other hand, argues that greater attention should be given to the "best interests of the child" in resolving disputes between birth and adoptive parents. She focuses on the impact of a custodial change on the child and questions the practice of dismissing an adoption proceeding and automatically transferring a child to a birth parent without taking into account the child's interests. She writes that even a fit birth parent's claims to custody may be limited because of a child's independent right to remain in the only custodial environment she has known [Hollinger 1995]. These conflicting views raise important questions about issues related to the meaning of parenthood and the nature of parent-child relationships in adoption. In disputes related to who is the "parent," who has primary status—the "biological" or "genetic" parent or the "social" parent? How should the concept of "best interests of the child" shape that determination?

The "Parent" in Assisted Reproduction

In assisted reproduction, disputes generally have centered on resolving the primacy of genetic or nongenetic parenthood (as in contested adoption cases), but importantly, unlike adoption, they also have focused on resolving the primacy of genetic or gestational parenthood. Courts frequently have given preference to genetic parentage, viewing nurturance and relationship-building as secondary to the genetic link between parent and child. As a consequence, genetically related adults, as opposed to nonrelated adults, generally prevail in child custody disputes [Mahoney 1995]. In assisted reproduction, however, the issues are often complicated by the presence of a gestational mother who carries a baby not genetically related to her. In some of these cases, the question is who of three women is the "real" mother: the woman who contributes her genetic material for the conception of the child, the woman who carries the child for nine months and then gives birth, or the woman who is the intended parent [Macklin 1991]. Courts are asked to determine which of these roles entitles a woman to a greater claim on the baby. Although courts have attempted to rely on legal principles in attempts to resolve this issue (as is the case in adoption), it may be, as Macklin [1991, p.

9] writes, that the question of who is the "real" mother to the offspring conceived through donor gametes is an ethical one involving a determination of "which factors are morally relevant and which have the greatest moral weight."

One perspective on the issue of "real" motherhood in assisted reproduction is that gestation is the determining factor. Annas [1988, p. 23], for example, argues that the gestational mother at the time of the child's birth has made the greatest personal contribution, a notion sometimes referred to as "sweat equity." The alternative justification for the emphasis on gestation is that the gestational mother has made the greatest "biological and psychological investment" in the child and she will, of necessity, be present at birth and immediately thereafter to care for the infant [Elias & Annas 1986, p. 67]. An opposing view is that motherhood is determined by genetics. From this perspective, the woman who makes the genetic contribution is the "mother," just as the inseminating male (as opposed to the husband of the woman who acts as a surrogate) is the "father" [Annas 1986, p. 31]. The alternative justification for this position is that children's best interests are served when their genetic parents rear them [Callahan 1987]. Finally, parenthood may be viewed primarily in terms of intent. Mead [1999, p. 63] notes that the "fertility industry" promotes the intentional view of parenthood, particularly through encouraging egg donors "to believe that what makes a woman into a mother is the wish to be a mother—to be what is known as...'the social parent.'" This perspective, however, has been subject to criticism. Mead [1999, p. 64], for example, questions the substitution of biological realities with the notion of parenting:

> A woman who bears an egg-donor child is encouraged to believe that carrying the fetus is the crucial component of motherhood. But a woman who hires a surrogate to carry her fertilized egg to term for her is encouraged to believe the opposite: that the important thing is the genetic link to the baby, and not the womb out of which the baby came. Biologically, an egg donor's situation is identical to that of a woman who uses a surrogate.

The major cases involving the competing claims of adults to a child conceived through assisted reproduction reflect the legal struggles to determine the primacy of genetics, gestation, or intent. In some cases, emphasis has been placed on the intent of parties regarding who will ultimately be the parents, although genetics has been a key, if not explicit, factor. In *Johnson v. Calvert* (1993), for example, a dispute arose between a gestational surrogate parent and the couple who were both the genetic (having contributed the egg and the sperm) and the intended parents of the child. The court ruled that the couple were the "real" parents of the child, ostensibly on the basis of their intent to parent. The court, however, seemed far more persuaded by the fact of the genetic tie that existed between the child and the intended parents. The court wrote that the surrogate's "role (was) as gestational host for the child (and) may be compared to that of a foster parent—she provided protection for the child during the period when its natural mother was unable to do so" [Cucci 1998, p. 424].

In the *Baby M* case, the dispute was between William and Elizabeth Stern, a couple who had entered into a contract with a surrogate with the intent that they would be the "parents," and the surrogate, Mary Beth Whitehead, who was both the genetic and gestational mother [Mahoney 1995]. The court, viewing the "unique legal arrangement" as nonetheless a contract, upheld the agreement and terminated Ms. Whitehead's parental rights, and allowed Mrs. Stern, the wife of the genetic father, to proceed with the adoption of the child [Mahoney 1995, p. 39]. The New Jersey Supreme Court, however, refused to sustain most of the trial court's rulings. The court declared surrogacy contracts, in general, to be equivalent to baby selling and declared the contract in issue to be unenforceable. The court, however, also allowed custody of the baby to remain with the Sterns on the basis of the child's "best interests," although at the same time, restoring Ms. Whitehead's parental rights and allowing her visitation with the child [Mahoney 1995]. The ruling by the New Jersey Supreme Court has been subject to widespread criticism [Gostin 1990; Smith 1990; Bezanson 1990]. Bezanson [1990, p. 247], for example, writes that:

The New Jersey Supreme Court should not have addressed the *Baby M* case in such a way to resolve, even by implication, the parentage and family issues raised by surrogacy. The court simply had no law on which to draw in resolving surrogacy's challenge to our society's moral and cultural view of maternity, paternity, and family.

The highly publicized case of a California couple, John and Luanne Buzzanca, illustrates courts' difficulties in determining who is *not* a parent in the context of assisted reproduction. In that case, the Buzzancas, finding that they were unable to conceive, obtained an embryo that had not been used in the course of IVF (and which was the result of a donor egg and the sperm of the infertile woman's husband). The Buzzancas enlisted the services of a gestational surrogate, and the embryo was transferred to her uterus. The couple's marriage, however, soured during the pregnancy. When a baby girl, Jaycee, was born, Luanne announced her plan to parent the baby, but John claimed that because he was neither the biological nor the legal father, he should not be required to pay child support. The trial court, although recognizing the roles that five adults (Mr. and Mrs. Buzzanca, the egg donor, the sperm donor, and the surrogate) had played in the child's birth, ruled that Jaycee had no legal parents. Subsequently, the California Court of Appeals reversed that decision, writing, "We disagree [with the trial court]. Let us get right to the point. Jaycee never would have been born had not Luanne and John both agreed to have a fertilized egg implanted in a surrogate" [cited in Andrews 1999]. The court declared that John's intent to be a parent was sufficient to hold him responsible for his child [Andrews 1999]. Litigation, however, continued and in yet a third ruling, a judge of the Orange County Superior Court released John from further support obligations to the then two-year old Jaycee, declared the surrogate contract unenforceable, and required Luanne to adopt Jaycee to finalize her parental rights [Vorzimer 1998]. Vorzimer [1998], taking issue with the court's rulings on a number of grounds, skeptically asks with regard to the need for Luanne's adoption of Jaycee, "Who then is Luanne supposed to adopt Jaycee from?"

Andrews [1999] points out that the variety of outcomes in the Buzzanca case, as well as other cases in which determinations of "parent" status in assisted reproduction have been made, illustrate the efforts of courts to fit the new reproductive technologies into existing laws. She [1999] further notes that "the pigeonholes that judges choose vary from state to state." When, for example, a surrogate mother decides to parent the child herself, some courts find analogues in adoption law (which allows birth mothers to reverse their consent) and rule in favor of the surrogate, and other courts apply contract law (relying on the terms of the original agreement between the parties) and rule in favor of the couple. As the Buzzanca case illustrates, courts can make a bewildering array of rulings that alternatively suggest the primacy of genetics in determining parenthood (the trial court and superior court rulings) and the primacy of intent to parent (the appellate court ruling).

Chapter 3

The Parties Served through Adoption and Assisted Reproduction

A focus on the parties served through adoption and assisted reproduction necessarily raises the question of who is the client in each of these services. Traditionally, adoption has been seen as a child welfare service that benefits, first and foremost, the child [Kirk 1964]. Assisted reproduction, by contrast, generally has been defined as a medical service that addresses the needs of infertile adults, with the primary client in egg, sperm, and embryo donation being the recipients of donor gametes [Greenfeld 1997; Sauer 1996]. The distinction between the traditional notion of adoption as a child-focused service and assisted reproduction as an adult-focused service, however, may be blurring, particularly in light of the market dynamics that currently characterize domestic infant adoption and international adoption practice (an issue that will be discussed later).

At the same time, issues arise about the interests and needs of the respective parties involved in adoption and donor conception. How do the interests of donors in assisted reproduction and birth parents in adoption compare? Are their roles similar or distinctly different? Are the interests of the child in adoption and the offspring conceived with donor gametes the same? Does explicit reliance on the principle of "best interests of the child" in adoption make that service meaningfully different than assisted reproduction where the interests of offspring are not expressly recognized? And finally, how do gamete recipients and prospective adoptive parents compare—particularly in relation to their access to the services they seek? Are the different approaches to gatekeeping in adoption and assisted reproduction appropriate?

Donors and Birth Parents

Birth parents in adoption and donors in assisted reproduction vary in their relationships to the parties who become the recognized parents. Birth parents may be relatives, friends, or strangers to the prospective adoptive parents. Similarly, donors may be related to recipients or may be unrelated and either known (or identified) or anonymous. Unlike birth parents in adoption, however, donors may be paid or altruistic. Although there is some research on birth parents' experiences (far more on birth mothers than birth fathers and far more on birth mothers who themselves place their children for adoption as opposed to birth mothers whose rights are involuntarily terminated), there is little research and, consequently, only limited understanding of the experiences of donors or the impact of donation on these individuals.

Over the past 20 years, research on adoption has led to a fuller understanding of the experiences of birth parents and has made clear that birth mothers and fathers do not easily move past their decisions to place their children for adoption nor do they forget the children they placed for adoption [Sorosky et al. 1984; Edwards 1995; Mason 1995]. Loss is an overarching theme in the psychological literature regarding the experiences of women who relinquish their children. This body of work suggests that loss is associated initially with the crisis pregnancy itself and that it deepens as the woman finds herself having to make a decision about her child, a process that is likely to evoke "feelings of denial, fear, anger, awe and outright panic" [Romanchik 1997, p. 2]. The clinical literature and the research suggest that the decision to relinquish a child for adoption also is likely to carry a sense of guilt and shame both at the time of and after the decision [Romanchik 1997].

The research further suggests that women who place their children for adoption are at significant risk of longer term physical, emotional, and interpersonal difficulties [Condon 1986; Edwards 1995; McHutchinson 1986; Van Keppel & Winkler 1983]. These studies indicate that many women who place their children for adoption suffer grief that continues over time [Van Keppel &

Winkler 1983]; experience ongoing problems in their relationships with family members and partners and difficulties in parenting subsequent children [Condon 1986]; adapt poorly or not at all
to placing their children for adoption [Bouchier et al. 1991]; and
often experience symptoms similar to posttraumatic stress disorder [Wells 1993].

Although there is only limited research on the impact of
adoption on birth fathers, studies suggest that rather than being
disinterested and desiring to flee all responsibility (the prevailing
stereotypes of birth fathers), birth fathers most often experience a
sense of uncertainty regarding the role they should play in a crisis
pregnancy [Mason 1995]. The uncertainty they feel typically
makes it difficult for them to play an active role in planning for the
child unless birth mothers welcome their participation [Mason
1995; Saunders 1996]. The research also indicates that although
birth fathers are typically viewed as unaccountable, irresponsible,
and absent during and after the pregnancy, most birth fathers, in
reality, have ongoing thoughts and concerns about their children
and do not forget them. Mason [1995, p. 15], for example, found
that although birth fathers often depersonalized the experience of
the pregnancy, birth, and planning for the child in order to
emotionally and physically distance themselves from pain and
uncertainty, every birth father she interviewed expressed a sense
of shame at not being able to assume the role of "dad."

There has been relatively little research involving sperm and
egg donors. As Berg [1995, p. 89] writes, "we do not understand
what it means to be a gamete donor—whether it is similar to
donating blood or a kidney, or is more like giving a child up for
adoption; and we particularly do not understand whether gender
differences exist in the psychology of donation." An understanding of donors, their decisions, and the impact of their decisions on
them has been limited by their relative invisibility, a reality that
in many ways corresponds to the historical status of birth parents
in adoption. Donor anonymity, which will be discussed in greater
detail later, has been the historical practice in assisted reproduction, and although this practice may be changing to some extent,

the environment of secrecy surrounding donors has resulted in their characterization as "types" rather than as "ethically significant figures with personal identities and moral characters" [Cohen 1996, p. 93]. Cohen [1996, p. 93] writes:

> [Donors] are taken into account instrumentally insofar as they affect the size of the donor pool and impinge on the welfare of recipients. When they are viewed as persons in their own right, they are seen as self-interested manipulators with little regard for their effect on the children born of their gametes or the recipient parents.

Typically, analogies between adoption and assisted reproduction have been drawn between birth parents and surrogates and not between birth parents and egg donors. Chesler [1988, cited in Macklin 1995], for example, warns of the dangers of surrogacy in light of the traumatic experiences of women who have relinquished their children for adoption. Ward [1988, cited in Macklin 1995, p. 298] likewise draws comparisons between the experiences of birth mothers and surrogates, pointing to "the sanctity of the bond between mother and child."

Ragoné's research with surrogate mothers [1996], however, suggests that such analogies may not apply. Ragoné found in her field research with surrogate mothers that "without exception, when surrogates are asked whether they think of the child as their own, they say that they do not" [1996, p. 360]. She also found that surrogates deemphasized their own link and biological contribution to the child and focused instead on the maternal role of nurturance. She [1996, p. 362] notes that:

> All the participants in the surrogate motherhood triad work to downplay the importance of the biological relatedness as it pertains to women...The idea that the adoptive mother [the spouse of the genetic father] is a mother by virtue of her role as nurturer is frequently echoed by all parties concerned. In this sense motherhood, as it pertains to surrogacy, is redefined as a social role.

These findings indicate that, at least in the short term, surrogates experience reproduction much differently than birth mothers.

Longer-term outcomes for surrogates, however, are not clear. Jean Benward [personal communication, June 26, 2000], for example, points to one study of surrogates who were interviewed ten years after the birth and who, as a group, expressed a high degree of dissatisfaction based on the nature of their relationships with the intended parents and the degree to which surrogates felt regarded and valued.

Similarities and differences in the role of egg donors and birth mothers have not been fully explored and warrant greater consideration. Jean Benward [personal communication, June 26, 2000] points out that egg donors are screened by mental health professionals and are selected for their ability to differentiate between "the egg" and the role of motherhood, and consequently, from the outset, the meaning that birth mothers and egg donors attribute to reproduction is markedly different. She [2000] also notes that there are likely to be significant differences between birth parents and egg donors in relation to the sense of voluntariness, choice, and attribution of control; that donors are less likely to feel shame and stigma than are birth mothers; and, at least in the short term, egg donors are more likely to be able to maintain an emotional detachment. She [2000] further points out, however, that it is not clear whether these distinctions between egg donors and birth mothers hold over time. It is not known whether over the long term, egg donors will experience loss and regret, nor is it clear the extent to which egg donors are psychically invested in their donor offspring. Women who "donate" their fertility desire intangible personal and psychological experiences as part of donation and may feel disappointment, loss, and regret when those experiences are not realized [Jean Benward, personal communication, June 26, 2000].

Analogies between adoption and assisted reproduction generally have not been made with regard to the men involved as sperm donors and birth fathers. The absence of attention to any potential similarities in men's experiences is somewhat ironic, given that much of the criticism directed toward birth fathers is that they function as little more than as sperm donors. Prager [1999, p. 363], for example, argues that birth fathers are simply men who "love their seed first" and not their children, a view shared by many who view birth fathers in functional terms and as essentially uninvolved, unconcerned and unaffected by outcomes involving their children [see Lightman & Schlesinger 1982]. Do sperm donors and birth fathers share common characteristics or experiences? Are their roles essentially the same or distinctly different?

Other equally important issues arise in relation to how sperm donors, egg donors, birth mothers and birth fathers are perceived by the professionals who serve them. To what extent are birth parents viewed as "clients" by adoption service providers and donors viewed as "patients" by medical professionals assisting infertile individuals? To the extent that they are clients or primary patients, how are their interests addressed? For example, is there fully informed consent for the decisions they are making? Do adoption service providers share with prospective birth parents what has been learned through research about the possible long-term psychological consequences of relinquishment? How do assisted reproduction professionals advise sperm and egg donors of the possible psychological and social consequences of their decisions, particularly given the limited understanding of these issues? Finally, when does the status of client or patient end? Does the acquisition of the gamete or the relinquishment of the child terminate professional responsibility to these parties and if so, what are the ethical implications of this practice? Little attention has been given to these issues, and as a consequence, they pose unresolved ethical questions bearing on the impact of both services on the individuals who essentially make the services possible.

Children and Offspring

There are varied perspectives on the extent to which adopted children and children conceived as a result of donor gametes have similar experiences. In reality, little is known about the impact of assisted reproduction on children, particularly those born as a result of egg, sperm, or embryo donation [Berg 1995]. Some assisted reproduction professionals, however, maintain that a child conceived from donor gametes does not face the same issues as an adoptee and that the two experiences should not be compared [see Golombok & Murray 1999]. Golombok and colleagues [1995, p. 297 (emphasis in original)], for example, draw distinctions between the psychological experiences of adoptees and offspring:

> It is important to point out...that while adoptive families and families with a child conceived by gamete donation are similar in that the child is genetically unrelated to at least one parent, the two types of families differ not only in that usually one parent *is* a genetic parent but also, and perhaps more importantly, in that the child had not been born to a genetically related mother and then given up for adoption. The fact that a child has always been a wanted child may constitute a very important difference.

These authors' emphasis on children's sense of "being wanted" as opposed to an understanding that they were "given up" poses important issues regarding longer-term outcomes for offspring and adoptees. Is the critical psychological distinction between adoptees and the offspring of donor gametes the sense of having "always been wanted" by the parents who rear them? Or is a sense of disconnection from genetic parents the key distinction? If, for example, a couple decides to donate their embryos after they have been preserved frozen for a number of years, would the offspring of these genetic parents feel—like adoptees—that they were "given up" by their "parents"?

Others contend that donor offspring are in effect "donor adoptees" and that they face similar issues as adopted children [Baran & Pannor 1989]. Baran and Pannor [1989], for example, argue that the offspring of donor gametes and adoptees have common experiences, particularly the "infantilizing" process that regards them as needing protection [Rowland 1985]. Some writers have attributed the lack of understanding of offspring experience to "the secrecy factor" in assisted reproduction [Sokoloff 1987, p. 15], and specifically, the fact that most donor offspring are not aware of their origins [Baran & Pannor 1989]. Sokoloff [1987, p.

15], in his review of the limited research on outcomes for offspring of assisted reproduction, suggests, however, that even offspring who have not been informed of the situation, have a general feeling of something being "off" in their families.

An increasingly recurrent theme in the literature is the lack of attention to the interests of the offspring of donor gametes. Freeman [1996 cited in Landau 1999, p. 194] observes that "assisted reproduction has hitherto neglected a children's rights perspective—and it shows it." Expressing a similar concern, Baran and Pannor [1989, p. 164] write that the "medical miracle" of assisted reproduction "is concentrated on fulfilling the needs of the infertile individual or couple; it allows no room for consideration of the lifelong effect on the child." Concerns about the lack of attention to the interests of offspring have been raised in relation to the decision-making of both gamete donors and recipients. Sokoloff [1987, p. 12], for example, contends that donors need to give far greater attention to the impact of their decisions on potential offspring:

> Is the anonymous (sperm) donor acting in the best interest of the child? Does he actually have adequate knowledge of his genetic background? Is he aware that he may be siring a substantial number of children in the same community, repetitively reproducing a genetic defect or creating a legitimate concern for future inbreeding?... The donor and physician each together have a choice and can guard their own interest. The child has none, and cannot.

Similarly, gamete recipients may not fully appreciate how their reproductive decision-making may impact their offspring in the longer term. Jean Benward [personal communication, June 26, 2000] points out that because recipients are desperate for a child and fearful of the genetic "other parent," they accept the role of secrecy in the use of donors gametes, and, similar to adoptive parents of previous generations, do not focus on the longer range impact of secrecy on the child's identity formation. Concerns continue to be expressed that non-disclosure will result in identity struggles and alienation for offspring, but the impact remains unclear and has not been the focus of research [Jean Benward, personal communication, June 26, 2000].

The lack of attention to the interests and needs of donor offspring in some ways parallels the pre-1970s inattention to the interests and needs of adoptees. In the 1970s with adoptees' organizational efforts that took the form of the Adoption Rights Movement, attention was brought to the impact of adoption practice and policy on adopted persons [Kuhns 1994; Carp 1992], and recently practice and policy have more fully addressed the concerns of these members of the triad [Gritter 1999a]. As Freeman [1996] notes, there has not as yet been a similar focus on the interests of offspring:

> There has been no systematic exploration of the questions [that assisted reproduction raises] which have put children, their interests and rights into the forefront... We owe the first generation of children of the reproductive revolution a better deal.

Because of the gap in understanding the experience of offspring, it is difficult to determine the extent to which offspring and adoptees have common interests and needs. It is clear that adoption, at least theoretically, is based on the concept of "best interests of the child," as will be discussed later. No such standard is utilized in relation to eggs or sperm, nor generally to embryos, though questions in this regard have arisen (also discussed later). The very different traditional child-centered focus of adoption as opposed to the adult-centered focus of assisted reproduction and the nature of each service (placement of an existing child versus services related to producing a potential child) highlight the difficulties in drawing comparisons between adoptees and offspring.

Prospective Adoptive Parents and Gamete Recipients

Issues also arise in relation to the interests and needs of prospective adoptive parents and the recipients of donor gametes. Although many considerations bear on the interests of these individuals, one key issue with ethical implications is the extent to which each group of prospective parents has access to the services they seek. Gatekeeping by professionals in terms of the screening of prospective adoptive parents historically has been a feature of adoption services. Professionals in assisted reproduction, however, traditionally have not viewed their role as one of controlling access to reproductive services or to parenthood. This distinction between assisted reproduction and adoption raises questions about the extent to which prospective parents should be required to qualify for parenting.

A key feature of adoption practice is the assessment of prospective adoptive parents for parental fitness. From a positive perspective, the assessment process (which generally involves a "home study") communicates to prospective families accurate information about adoption; provides prospective families with the opportunity to determine their suitability as adoptive parents by identifying their own strengths and vulnerabilities; and prepares families for the challenges of parenting an adopted child [Rycus et al. 1998]. It also provides a basis for assuring birth parents that care is being taken in placing their children with appropriate adoptive families [Jean Benward, personal communication, June 26, 2000]. Assessment for purposes of adoption, however, has generated criticism as "the only screening for parenthood sanctioned in our society" [Lieberman 1998, p. 4]. Hollinger [1985], for example, has pointed to a number of deficiencies in the assessment process, including reliance on stereotypes as to who is a "fit" parent and the use of subjective measures of fitness. Prospective adoptive parents typically describe the assessment process as a "daunting" experience involving a "passive and sometimes threatening process over which they [have] little control" [Clark et al. 1998, p. 35]. Barker and colleagues [1998, p. 2] similarly characterize the process as "an obstacle course" in which applicants must "jump through hoops," give the "right" answers to validate themselves as individuals and as potential parents, and convince those with power, social workers within agencies, to allow them to parent.

By contrast, individuals generally are not screened for parental fitness in assisted reproduction [see Andrews 1998], and parental screening is not viewed as relevant to the needs of offspring or donors [J. Benward, personal communication, June 26, 2000]. Some have criticized the absence of screening of individuals as prospective parents before they are provided with assisted reproduction services [Andrews 1998]. In some states, legislation has been proposed to require counseling of any party seeking any form of alternative reproduction, but such efforts have not been successful [Andrews 1998]. To the extent that parental assessment in the assisted reproductive context does occur, it is only under very limited circumstances and is mandated by the courts, not utilized as part of the process of providing assisted reproduction. Andrews [1998] indicates, for example, that in surrogacy cases, the nongenetic intended mother is generally required to adopt the child, and, in some cases, courts have relied on adoption law and ordered a full investigation of the suitability of both intended parents. Such assessments, however, are not ordered when a surrogate serves as the gestational mother only, and the embryo is genetically related to both intended parents [Andrews 1998].

The question arises as to whether screening for parental fitness is appropriate in assisted reproduction. Andrews [1998, p. 14-37] notes that "the screening for suitability to parent may be thought of as a substitute for the biological bond in determining who should be allowed to raise children." On the basis of that rationale, she [1998] contends that there is no need for screening when one or both of the intended parents has a genetic connection with the child as the biological tie sufficiently establishes parental merit. In cases, however, in which there is no genetic tie between the child and either intended parent, the biological proof of parental sufficiency is absent. Would these situations suggest the need for parental assessment? Screening in cases of embryo donation or the combined use of egg and sperm donation, for example, could be justified on the basis of the adoption model as the substitute for the genetic tie. Objections to screening even in these cases, however, may still be raised. Andrews [1998, p. 14-37,

14-38], for example, writes that "screening opens up the possibility for an abuse of discretion whereby people who would be good parents are nonetheless denied the opportunity because they are thought not to be socially desirable." This objection, which lies at the heart of much of the criticism of prospective parent assessment in adoption, suggests that screening may be entirely too arbitrary to function effectively.

A number of questions remain to be resolved in the context of screening for parental fitness in both adoption and assisted reproduction. Is the adoption model of parental assessment the appropriate approach to ensure suitability for parenthood? Should home studies be conducted of prospective parents seeking assisted reproduction? Or, alternatively, is the assisted reproduction model the sounder approach, allowing access to parenthood by all who desire services and can pay for assistance? Does the answer depend ultimately on who is defined as the client—the adults who seek and purchase the service or the child/offspring who is sought?

Chapter 4

Anonymity and Information Access

One of the key dilemmas currently confronting assisted reproduction and adoption is the extent to which information should be shared among the parties involved in each service. Benward and Asch [1999] pose the question that lies at the basis of issues related to anonymity and information sharing as: "Can we formulate policy that grants legitimacy to the offspring's desire to know, to develop a coherent sense of self, while recognizing that a family is more than 'blood' ties and families formed through non-coital reproduction and adoption require legitimacy as well?"

In adoption, practices related to secrecy have changed dramatically over the past 10 to 15 years. In the early part of the twentieth century, information about birth parents was non-existent or minimal, as information was rarely recorded and the information that was available was often inaccurate [Freundlich & Peterson 1998]. Beginning in the 1950s, information was collected to a greater degree but disclosure tended to be selective, with generally only positive information about a child shared with prospective adoptive parents [Freundlich & Peterson 1998]. Under current practice, health, social, and other information about birth parents is collected to a far greater extent and non-identifying information is generally made available to both adoptive parents and adult adoptees [Freundlich & Peterson 1998]. At the same time, practice has shifted so that birth parents often are involved in selecting the adoptive parents for their children and typically receive background information on prospective families in order to make an informed choice of a family for their children [Modell 1994].

Access by adult adoptees to identifying information regarding their birth parents, however, is an issue that continues to be hotly contested. On the one hand, clinical literature has high-

lighted the psychological impact on adoptees of having no or only
uncertain information about their birth parents and has associated
lack of such information with confusion, uncertainty, and other
negative effects on adoptees' sense of self and psychological well-
being [Rowland 1985, p. 391 citing Sants 1964]. On the other hand,
it is asserted that adoptees generally fare well psychologically,
and that information about birth parents is not only unnecessary
but can be affirmatively harmful to them [Byrd 1998].

Like traditional adoption, assisted reproduction has been
marked by "secrecy and anonymity" [Benward & Asch 1999].
Because of the stigma attached to sperm donation (the earliest
form of gamete donation), virtual anonymity has been the traditional practice. Historically, information on sperm donors, including donor medical histories, was not collected at all or only
minimally, and even when collected in more complete form, was
destroyed after a short period of time [Asche 1985]. Donors'
identities were not made known, and donors usually were not
made aware of the reproductive outcomes associated with their
donations. Similar to the rationales for complete confidentiality
in adoption, anonymity in sperm donation grew out of the desire
to protect the privacy of recipients and family; unlike adoption,
there also was a desire to protect donors against future financial
responsibilities for offspring and to protect the doctor from "social
condemnation and legal liability" [Benward 1998, p. 1].

The practice of complete secrecy in assisted reproduction,
however, has changed to some degree, particularly in the arena of
sperm donation. In the late 1980s, the advent of AIDS and federal
recommendations that all donor inseminations utilize frozen
quarantined semen precipitated several changes: more complete
collection of information on sperm donors, disclosure of information to recipients, and more extensive record keeping [Benward &
Asch 1999]. With quarantine of sperm and the creation of sperm
banks as an alternative to physicians' collection of donated sperm,
detailed record keeping became the norm [Benward 1998]. Sperm
banks now generally collect fairly comprehensive information
from and maintain records on donors; some offer photos and
videotapes of donors for recipients to review; and there is growing

support for the practice of providing identifying information on donors to offspring [Benward & Asch 1999; Rowland 1985].

In contrast to the long-standing practice of anonymity in programs for sperm donors, egg donation began "almost exclusively with known donors" [Braverman 1993, p. 1219]. Given the initial technology of egg donation, few women were willing to undergo egg extraction on behalf of strangers, and, as a result, women who donated eggs typically had personal relationships with recipients [Cohen 1996]. As egg donation evolved and the risks decreased with the advent of new technologies, however, anonymous donors became more common [Cohen 1996]. In contrast to the trend away from anonymity in sperm donation, greater allegiance to anonymity in egg donation has developed [Cohen 1996]. Currently, many egg donation programs practice anonymous donation only, and psychologists and nurses make the "match" between recipients and donors [Mead 1999]. Much as was the case in adoption prior to the 1990s when social workers matched adoptive parents and children without any involvement of birth parents, donors are not given information on recipients and recipients do not meet donors or even see pictures of the women whom the program has chosen as donors for them [Mead 1999]. Additionally, in contrast to the current practice of providing recipients with significant background information on sperm donors, the disclosure of non-identifying background information on egg donors has continued to vary widely [Benward 1998].

Issues related to sharing or withholding information in assisted reproduction arise in several contexts, as is the case in adoption. These issues center on disclosure of the use of assisted reproduction as the form of family formation and the disclosure of both non-identifying and identifying information on donors to recipients and offspring.

Disclosure of the Use of Assisted Reproduction

There are key issues related to disclosing to others that the family was formed through assisted reproduction, and, perhaps more importantly, disclosing to the child the facts related to her genetic origins. It is now common that families alert friends and families of their intention to adopt, although such a decision was carefully guarded in earlier times (the 1950s through the early 1970s) because of the social stigma that surrounded the adoption of children not of "one's blood" and prevailing social attitudes that adoptive families were not "normal" [Gill in press]. It appears that similar social stigmas may surround the formation of families through assisted reproduction and support greater secrecy in this regard.

Klock and Maier [1991], for example, found in their study that recipients of donor gametes resisted disclosing information about their use of assisted reproduction and that those who did disclose regretted doing so. The researchers found that 81% of parents who had had a child with the assistance of donor insemination reported that if it were possible to go back and do it over again, they would not disclose the nature of the pregnancy to others. "Regret about others knowing about a donor may result because the family does not wish to be seen as 'different,' once they have adapted to parenthood" [Braverman 1999, p. 8]. Others argue, however, that support for secrecy in this regard undermines truthfulness as a significant social value [Cohen 1996]. Daniels and Taylor [1993, p. 159], for example, argue that "it is the generally accepted norm in social relations that openness and truthfulness are to be preferred," and if an exception is to be made for assisted reproduction, "the arguments against openness and truth-telling must be carefully examined to determine if such an exception is specifically justified."

Of equal, if not greater, importance is the extent to which information about a child's genetic origin should be communicated to the child who is created through assisted reproduction. Adoptive parents commonly are advised to tell their children they were adopted, and adoptive parents typically do so [Melina 1986]. Such has not been the practice in assisted reproduction. The majority of parents report that they are not likely to tell their children of their genetic parentage, and among those who initially plan to do so, many later change their minds and withhold the information from their children [Blyth 1999; Golombok 1997; Klock et al. 1994]. Cook and associates [1994] compared the level of disclosure to children by donor insemination parents, in vitro fertilization parents, and adoptive parents. The researchers found that none of the parents who conceived via donor insemination and only 27% of the parents who conceived through in-vitro fertilization had told their children about their origins, whereas all but one of the adopted children knew that he or she had been adopted. Golombok and Murray [1999], in their study of donor insemination parents, similarly found that all the parents who had used sperm donation and all but one of the parents who had used egg donation had decided not to provide any information to their children about their genetic parentage, with the greatest commitment to secrecy in families in which the father was the nongenetic parent. The researchers found, however, that one-half of the parents who had used sperm donation and almost three-quarters who had used egg donation had shared this information with persons other than the child, suggesting that the information may not remain secret despite the intent to withhold the information from the child.

As the research suggests, it is still the case that the majority of children conceived by gamete donation are not told about their origins [Amuzu et al. 1990; Braverman 1999; Klock & Maier 1991]. The practice of recommending to parents that they keep the use of a donor secret from their child, however, has become subject to greater debate [Braverman 1999]. Parents increasingly are being encouraged to disclose to their children information about their genetic histories [Daniels & Lewis 1996], but many family therapists express ambivalence about the benefits of such disclosure to children and urge that disclosure be decided on a case by case basis [Chasin 1993]. Resistance to disclosure appears based on convictions that explaining to a child her origins is "irrelevant to the child" [Cook et al. 1994, p. 553]; uncertainties about the age when parents should tell their children; and concerns about how parents should tell their children given the complexities of the treatment process [Cook, et al. 1994].

Disclosure of Donor Information

A second issue relates to nonidentifying and identifying information about donors and the disclosure of each type of information to recipients and to offspring. To some extent, research has addressed these issues through surveys of donors regarding their attitudes about the disclosure of both types of information and the extent to which such disclosure would affect their willingness to donate. In two studies, one conducted in New Zealand and one in Houston, Texas, researchers found that 90% of sperm donors were willing to provide personal information about themselves, including medical and psychosocial histories, so that the information could be shared with recipients [Andrews 1998]. The majority of donors believed that such information was important to the well-being of potential offspring. Almost 60% of the donors stated that they would agree to personal contact when offspring reached the age of 18 or older [Andrews 1998]. When donors in the Houston program were asked if they would donate if anonymity were not guaranteed, more than 80% stated that they would be donors under such circumstances [Andrews 1998].

Earlier studies, however, reveal somewhat greater ambivalence among sperm donors about their willingness to donate if identifying information were shared. In a study described by Rowland [1985], 67 sperm donors were surveyed about their views of anonymity. The majority (82%) stated that they were willing to provide non-identifying information, and more than half of the donors stated that they would not mind if "their offspring contacted them after the age of 18" [Rowland 1985, p. 394]. Only 42% of donors, however, stated that they would donate if anonymity were not guaranteed. In another study of the attitudes of 79 sperm donors, Mahlstedt and Probasco [1991] found that the majority of donors (90%) were willing to provide detailed medical, social, educational, and personal histories and virtually all of the donors (96%) were willing to have the information shared with recipient families in a non-identifying form. Substantially fewer donors (about 37%), however, were willing to have full identifying information shared.

With regard to disclosure of medical, psychosocial and other background information on donors, the extent of disclosure inevitably will be affected by practices related to collection of information and donor screening. Medical and psychological screening and counseling appear to vary significantly among programs, "although there appears to be a consensus and general acceptance of the role of both" [Braverman 1993, p. 1219]. Screening of sperm donors has become extensive, with many clinics utilizing a four-generation family medical history of parents, grandparents, and siblings; the donor's sexual history, including any risky behaviors; a comprehensive physical examination, including a semen and blood analysis to screen for abnormalities or diseases; and for repeat donors, regular laboratory testing and updates of family medical histories twice a year [Braverman 1993]. Psychological screening and counseling of sperm donors, however, are not the norm [Jean Benward, personal communication, June 26, 2000].

There appears to be even greater variation in the practices of egg donor programs related to information collection. Braverman [1993] found that although 93% of the egg donation programs surveyed over a seven month period tested for human immunodeficiency virus (HIV), only 7% tested for drug use and 21% did not conduct physical examinations of egg donors. Although 78% of the surveyed programs conducted psychological evaluations of donors, only 60% utilized established criteria for donor acceptance or rejection based on psychological testing results. In this connection, Braverman [1993, p. 1220] notes that increasingly greater attention is being given by egg donation programs to "expectations and procedures of psychological and medical evaluations and education" for egg donors in order to "improve the current practice of ovum donor programs [in meeting] the needs of both donors and recipients." The American Society for Reproductive Medicine [2000], in its guidelines, includes recommendations for medical and psychological screening of egg donors. Nonetheless, as Andrews [1998] points out, some infertility specialists continue to maintain that because individuals do not screen one another for medical and genetic factors before they have a biological child, screening of donors is likewise neither necessary nor desirable.

The increased attention to the medical, genetic and psychosocial histories of donors parallel developments in adoption, where over the last decade adoption agencies increasingly have confronted issues related to obtaining and disclosing information to prospective adoptive families about the health and social background of children and their birth families. Although quality practice supports the sharing of such information, litigation brought by adoptive parents in this regard has shown that, in a number of cases, adoption agencies and independent practitioners have failed to provide prospective adoptive families with known information about a child's physical, emotional or developmental problems or with critical background information about the child's birth family and history. In these cases, adoptive families, deprived of such information, have found themselves neither emotionally nor financially prepared to care for a child whose needs require enormously expensive medical or mental health treatment, and they have initiated law suits to recover the costs of their children's care [Freundlich & Peterson 1998].

In response to litigation initiated by adoptive families, courts have recognized a duty to disclose known material information about a child's health and social background to prospective adoptive families. In the face of a breach of the duty to disclose, courts have held agencies liable for the tort of "wrongful adoption" and awarded adoptive families monetary damages. An agency's breach of the duty to disclose can take many forms and, depending on the state, liability may be imposed when agencies misrepresent a child's background, deliberately withhold information, or are negligent in providing prospective adoptive parents with information that could be material to their decision whether to adopt a particular child [Freundlich & Peterson 1998].

Similar legal issues are beginning to surface in assisted reproduction. In a recent case, a California court ruled that an anonymous donor did not have an unlimited right to privacy and could, in fact, be forced to testify in a legal action that alleged that his sperm caused genetic harm to the child that he helped to be conceived [CNN 2000]. The sperm bank resisted the family's efforts to obtain information on the donor, unsuccessfully arguing that anonymity was essential: "If the donor doesn't believe it's confidential, [he] might not donate" [CNN 2000]. In rejecting this argument, the court placed primary weight on the importance of donors' health and genetic information in relation to the well-being of offspring, even to the extent of mandating the disclosure of the identity of a donor who wished to remain anonymous. Should the law continue to develop along this line, paralleling the tort of wrongful adoption, service providers may be required to place greater emphasis on the collection and disclosure of background information on donors.

Access to Identifying Information and Search

Although it appears that some number of adoptees wish to obtain identifying information about their birth parents [Hartman & Laird 1990; Lifton 1994; Sorosky et al. 1984] and search for members of their birth families [Auth & Zaret 1986; Triseliotis 1973], it is not clear to what extent donor offspring desire to obtain information about their genetic origins or contact their genetic parents. Issues surrounding loss—which characterize the experiences of many adoptees and lead them to search for members of their birth families to understand why they were placed for adoption [Modell 1994]—may not be relevant concerns for donor offspring. Reitz and Watson [1992, p. 237], for example, outline as one of the major reasons for adoptees' decisions to search, "the need to know why they were abandoned to adoption." There may, however, be other reasons for searching that adoptees and donor offspring share. Research in adoption, for example, suggests that adoptees search because they have the desire to "find out who I really am," "learn my true identity," and find "the part of me that is missing" [Schechter & Bertocci 1990, p.80]. It may be that offspring have similar interests related to their genetic identities, which may precipitate efforts to contact the donors who contributed to their conceptions. The extent to which offspring have such interests is not known, however, beyond anecdotal accounts.

The circumstances surrounding search and reunion are likely to be different, at least in some regards, in adoption and assisted reproduction. One critical difference between the two types of searches is the nature of the birth parent's and the donor's role. In an adoption-related search, a birth parent may be contacted by his or her only birth child, whereas in assisted reproduction, a sperm donor may be responsible for 20 or more offspring, each of whom may have a desire for a connection with his or her genetic father [Benward & Asch 1999]. Although the interest in locating genetic parents conceivably may be no different for an adoptee and an offspring of donor gametes, the outcomes of such searches may be quite different for the genetic parents. The fact that donors may make multiple gamete donations (as opposed to contributing to the birth of a single child) raises a host of issues related to release of identifying information and search as well as other issues regarding the number of offspring to whom an individual should be allowed to genetically contribute.

The Differing Perspectives on Disclosure

The rights of offspring in relation to access to information about themselves is a key issue in assisted reproduction, just as it has been a key issue in adoption. Morrison [2000, p. 14] notes that although donor assisted conception is on the rise, "unlike adopted or surrogate children, these children have no rights under the law to obtain information about their origins." He [2000, p. 14] contends that although donors may desire the reassurance of anonymity (or, in the case of sperm donors, the distance of "remote fathering"), there may be highly negative consequences for offspring when information is withheld. In language reminiscent of debates in adoption regarding the importance of genetic information, Morrison [2000, p. 14] observes:

> Scientifically, fertilisation and embryology may be a brave new world. But ethically, they belong to the old

Victorian shadowland of secrets and lies...Until we can conceive humans who have no interest in their genes, until identity itself is annulled and de-historicised, there will always be someone who wants to know.

The arguments made in favor of and against disclosure of information to the offspring of third party reproduction parallel those made in adoption. Arguments in favor of disclosure generally rest on experiences from adoption that suggest that children fare better when family origins are discussed openly. The major arguments advanced in support of disclosure in assisted reproduction include:

- Individuals have a fundamental right to know about their genetic origins [Baran & Pannor 1989; Braverman 1999];

- Medical information is critical, and non-disclosure limits the amount of information that the child receives [Braverman 1999];

- Secrets are lethal and may permanently hurt the child and the family [Baran & Pannor 1989];

- Children born through donor gametes will sense, through subtle cues, that there is something "different" about themselves, with resulting negative effects on their sense of self and their relationships with their families [Baran & Pannor 1989; Braverman 1999]; and

- Disclosure helps to eliminate the odds of related individuals marrying one another, particularly given the frequency of donations by some donors [Lamport 1988.]

In line with these arguments, some donor offspring have joined together to advocate for greater access to information. The Donor Conception Support Group of Australia, for example, was established by donor offspring and their recipient parents in an effort to promote greater access by offspring to full information about their genetic parents [South Australian Council on Reproductive Technology 2000]. In this regard, Rowland [1985, pp. 931-932] contends that:

> Currently, we are...committing the same error which those in control of adoption previously committed...We always refer to them as children, thus allocating to ourselves the right to decide what is best for them. But like adoptees, offspring will eventually be adults...who will have definite opinions about their rights.

On the other hand, arguments are advanced to support confidentiality of information in assisted reproduction. These contentions also parallel the arguments made in favor of closed or confidential adoptions:

- Individuals do not have a fundamental right to know about their genetic origins and their interest in obtaining more information fails to supercede the donor's wish for anonymity;

- Medical information can be effectively incorporated into the child's and the family's medical history to ensure accurate information without disclosing further information;

- All families have secrets, and every day parents choose what information to tell or not tell their children;

- Children will be socially stigmatized if information is revealed about their genetic origins;

- Children born through donor gametes will not sense anything different when their parents are loving and are not conflicted about the use of donor gametes;

- Anonymity protects families from interference or harassment from donors and protects donors' privacy within their own families;

- Sperm donation has taken place under restrictions of confidentiality for years, and the families involved appear to have managed well;

- Should donors be encouraged to reveal their identities, they would be less inclined to donate; and

- From a religious and moral perspective, secrecy supports the uniqueness of the marital relationship and acknowledges the particular sensitivity that must be paid to the issue of male infertility [Blyth 1999; Braverman 1999; Cohen 1996; Cook et al. 1994].

Some commentators also urge that the lessons learned from adoption regarding anonymity, secrecy, and disclosure are not necessarily appropriate in assisted reproduction. Klock and colleagues [1994, p. 482], for example, write that, "we cannot assume that the accepted guidelines for adoption are always applicable to every family formed using donor insemination. Decisions regarding disclosure must be made by the recipient couple in the context of their own lives." Golombok [1997, pp. 378-379] similarly urges a consideration of the similarities and differences between "the donor gamete child" and an adopted child in assessing the benefits and risks of disclosure:

The donor gamete child who is aware of his/her donor origin faces many of the same issues as an adopted child, including (i) being raised by at least one non-biologically related parent, (ii) having some understanding that he/ she is "different" from other children; (iii) at times rejecting his/her non-biological parent; and (iv) wanting more information about the donor, the "missing" parent.

Alternatively, the donor gamete child is different from an adopted child in several important ways, including (i) having a genetic connection to one recipient parent, (ii) his/her gestation and delivery occurring in the context of the recipients' relationship, (iii) not being "given up" or "surrendered" by the biological parents, and (iv) being aware of the general lack of societal approval of donor gamete use as a means of family building.

The "donor gamete child" who is conceived through combined sperm and egg donation or, alternatively, through embryo donation, would not have the genetic connection to one parent that Golombok notes and, at least in connection with embryo donation, may have a sense of being "given up" by the biological parents. It is as yet unclear whether these distinctions cause donor offspring to more closely resemble adoptees in psychological and social terms than do children of other types of assisted reproduction.

Policies on Disclosure of Donor Information

In the United States, there are no uniform policies on disclosure of information about donors in assisted reproduction. A few countries, however, have developed such policies, with varying approaches taken to the benefits and risks of information disclosure. In Great Britain, the Feversham Committee [1960, p. 59, cited in Blyth 1999, pp. 49-50] observed in 1960 that semen donation was "an activity which might be expected to attract more than the usual proportion of psychopaths," and concluded, as a result, that there were important reasons that anyone involved in assisted reproduction keep their participation "a closely guarded secret." The Committee determined that the best interests of children born as a result of such procedures would be served by never revealing to the children the nature of their births [Blyth 1999]. In 1987, however, the Warnock Committee reversed the practice of secrecy in semen donor conception when it concluded that secrecy served to "undermine the whole network of family relationships" and determined that it was "wrong to deceive children about their origins" [Department of Health and Social Security 1984, p. 15]. The Warnock Committee recommended that offspring have access to the donors' medical and ethnic background information when they reached the age of eighteen.

The Warnock Committee's recommendations provided the basis for Great Britain's Human Fertilisation and Embryology Act enacted in 1990. Under the Act, licensed infertility centers are required to maintain records of donors, recipients of donated gametes and embryos, and children born following treatment, and they are required to forward this information to the statutory regulatory body, the Human Fertilisation and Embryology Authority (HFEA) for inclusion on the Register of Information. HFEA advises infertility centers to encourage sperm donors "to provide as much...non-identifying biographical information about themselves as they wish, to be made available to prospective parents and any resulting child" [HFEA 1998, p.23]. Although these requirements allow access to information, they do not ensure, as Blyth [1999] points out, that information will be disclosed nor do they guarantee the accuracy of the information that is conveyed.

In contrast to the British approach, legislation in three countries—Sweden, Austria and Australia [Victoria]—unequivocally gives donor offspring the right to learn the identity of the donor [Blyth 1999]. The Infertility Act of 1995 of Victoria, Australia, which took effect in 1998, is the most comprehensive of such legislation. Recognizing that donor offspring become adults, the legislation specifically states that "the welfare and interests of any person born or to be born as a result of a treatment procedure are paramount" and makes explicit the right of offspring to access information about their genetic origins [cited in Blyth 1999, p. 55.] At age 18, donor offspring may obtain both nonidentifying and identifying information about the donor. The Act also specifically recognizes that recipients of donated gametes have the right, with the donor's consent, to learn the donor's identity and provides that with the consent of recipients or donor offspring at age 18, donors may learn the identity of the offspring.

These differing legislative approaches in some ways resemble the divergent state law approaches in the United States to adult adoptees' access to identifying information regarding their birth parents. The legal approaches used in the adoption context reflect efforts to address some of the very concerns that have surfaced in other countries' policies regarding the access of offspring to information on donors. State laws in the U.S. governing adult adoptees' access to identifying information on their birth parents attempt to balance the various interests of adoptees, birth parents, and adoptive parents through three major approaches: (1) release of identifying information upon a showing to a court of "good cause" (which requires a court to determine a compelling need for such information) [Kuhns 1994; Hollinger 1999b]; (2) release upon mutual registration on a designated registry in which identifying information is released only when both the birth parent and adult adoptee file formal consents to the disclosure of their identities [Avery 1996]; and (3) release upon engaging a "confidential intermediary" to locate a birth parent on behalf of an adult adoptee (or vice versa) and the third party's determination that the birth parent or adoptee is willing to disclose his or her identity or meet the other party [Avery 1996]. Currently in only five states do adult adoptees have direct and unconditional access to their original birth certificates—Kansas, Alaska, Tennessee, Alabama, and Oregon [Cloud 2000]. As the debates around the changes in the "closed records" laws in Tennessee and Oregon, however, demonstrate [Trevison 1997; Verhovek 2000], there is considerable resistance to allowing adult adoptees to access identifying information on their birth parents. The tensions surrounding this issue in adoption reflect the ongoing concerns in this area.

Similarly, although the collection and maintenance of information on donors are of growing interest, "the issues surrounding the release of information continue to be controversial" [Benward 1998, p. 9]. Some commentators urge that "donors must provide recipients, and ultimately the resulting children, with relevant information that may be carried in this genetic material" [Cohen 1996, p. 95]. Others contend that the obligation of the donor goes beyond genetic and medical information and extends to moral duties as a "parent" [Cohen 1996]. These issues again raise questions about the essence of parenthood as biological or social, as discussed earlier. As Crockin [1999, p. 473] notes,

> Collaborative reproduction, in the form of sperm, egg, and embryo donation...by challenging our established notions of biological and legal parentage and opening the door to increased anonymous, commercialized

reproduction...create significant legal, ethical, and societal issues needing to be resolved that reach far
beyond the private decisions of providers and their
adult patients.

Chapter 5

Market Forces in Adoption and Assisted Reproduction

Market forces have become increasingly apparent in both the adoption of infants and in assisted reproduction. The fees associated with each service have reached significant levels, and to a growing extent, only those individuals with meaningful resources have access to services. Recipients of donor gametes and those seeking to become adoptive parents of healthy infants generally have a level of resources that exceeds those of donors or birth parents and, consequently, are perceived as having greater power in the relationships on which the services are based [Freundlich 2000]. At the same time, individuals within both groups of potential parents—because they are, in Gritter's words [1999b], the "paying customers"—have demonstrated increasingly specific expectations regarding the age, health, ethnicity, and other characteristics of the child they wish to parent. These features of infant adoption suggest that the traditional child-centered focus of adoption has begun to erode, and, at least in relation to domestic infant adoption, emphasis may have shifted to serving prospective parents as the primary clients. That focus suggests a similarity to the service emphasis in assisted reproduction where medical services are unquestionably adult-focused. The rise in adoption fees, the discrepancies found in the "price" to be paid to adopt children of different races and ethnicities, and the willingness of some families to pay higher fees for children who physically resemble them further suggest that from a market perspective, infant adoption and assisted reproduction may closely resemble one another.

The Role of Money in Adoption and Assisted Reproduction

Money has come to play a significant role in both adoption and assisted reproduction. In adoption, there is the question of the propriety of any payment whatsoever. Watson [1999], for example, argues that fees charged prospective adoptive parents are not appropriate under any circumstances because they raise the potential for financial exploitation and cannot be justified as anything other than payment for a child. Specifically, he takes issue with the argument that fees cover "services," pointing to the widely varying definitions of what constitutes "services to adoptive parents," a variation that he maintains "is based less on the quality of agency service than on the fiscal base of an agency and how it calculates its fees" [Watson 1999, p. 7]. That said, however, there is general agreement that at least some costs associated with adoption represent actual expenses connected with the provision of services (home studies, birth parent counseling services, and legal services) and must be met in some way. If, indeed, payment at some level for some purpose in adoption is acceptable, the question then becomes how much should be paid and what actually is being purchased.

Similar questions arise in assisted reproduction. The significant costs often associated with assisted reproduction, in general, and the practice of paying for eggs and for surrogacy services, in particular, have given rise to a host of ethical questions [Robertson 1988-89; Arneson 1992]. Should donors be paid for sperm or eggs? Is the practice of paying surrogates acceptable? And, if payment itself is appropriate, what level of payment is acceptable?

Money and Adoption

The cost of adopting a healthy infant currently ranges from $10,000 to $20,000, though it is not uncommon for individuals to pay as much as $30,000 or more for a healthy Caucasian infant [Jacoby 1999; Pertman 1998]. Dramatically larger figures are at times reported in connection with independently arranged adoptions through attorneys, with reports that some prospective adoptive parents have paid as much as $100,000 in order to adopt a newborn [Mansnerus 1998]. The willingness to pay amounts significantly greater than average agency fees reflects, in large part, the desire—and the financial ability—of prospective adoptive parents to move to the head of the waiting line and adopt a healthy Caucasian infant in a relatively short period of time [see Freundlich 2000].

There is general agreement that the amount of money involved and the potential for making money in infant adoption have greatly increased since the 1960s. Watson [1999, p. 7] attributes this trend to three key factors: the availability of fewer infants for adoption as a result of legal and social changes; "the growing belief that everything in our country (health, information, peace of mind, children) is a commodity that can be packaged, marketed and sold at a profit;" and the ability of an increasing number of affluent young adults who are willing to pay whatever is required to satisfy their desire to become parents. These factors suggest that the escalation in the amount of money involved in infant adoption is the result of the combined effects of diminished supply, an adult sense of entitlement, and affluence, factors which might also be attributed to the market dynamics of assisted reproduction.

Considerable criticism has surfaced with regard to the rising costs of adoption. Some assert that prospective adoptive parents are being exploited by the increasing fees they are required to pay in order to adopt; others maintain that prospective adoptive parents themselves have created the environment in which higher fees can be charged, with the most affluent, consequently, benefiting [Freundlich 2000]. Concerns also focus on the extent to which the increasing sums of money associated with the adoption of infants impact birth parents, particularly their decision-making regarding adoption [Gritter 1999b]. When birth parents are provided with significant financial support (an issue discussed later), there is the reality that they may be reluctant to decide later that they wish to parent their child themselves, even when they believe strongly that adoption is not the right choice for them

[Gritter 1999b]. Gritter [1999b, p. 11] notes that "another worrisome possibility is that expectant birth parents may exploit the desperation of prospective adoptive parents by misleading them about their intentions." Finally, in considering the increasing role of money in adoption, the question has become whether infants have been transformed into commodities, rated on the basis of age, race, gender, health, physical attractiveness, or other desired characteristics, and available to those individuals who are able to pay the highest fee [Freundlich 2000]. This issue is discussed later in greater detail.

Money and Assisted Reproduction

As with market dynamics in infant adoption, money is seen as playing a key role in assisted reproduction in general, and as driving the quest for donor eggs in particular. Money has become an issue at two levels: the overall costs of assisted reproduction for the recipients of services and the fees paid to gamete donors. As Macklin and White [1997] point out, there is considerable disagreement about the exchange of money for gametes in assisted reproduction. Some argue that paying for gametes does not necessarily translate into a negative practice; others, however, contend that "transactions involving money represent a form of commercialization and commodification" and that exchanges of money for human eggs (but, interestingly, not sperm) and payments to surrogates "should be blocked" [Macklin & White 1997, p. 130].

Total costs for assisted reproduction vary, depending on the service that is utilized and the number of services received. Couples undergoing in vitro fertilization generally pay fees in the range of $8,000 to $10,000 per cycle, with many couples requiring multiple cycles to achieve a birth [Greenfeld 1997]. Collins and associates [1995] report that in 1993, the computed cost of a live birth from in vitro fertilization was more than $40,000, although others state that this estimate is conservative, with the average cost actually ranging from $66,667 to $114,286, depending on the number of cycles utilized [Neumann, Gharib & Weinstein 1994]. With regard to egg donation, the average cost of in vitro fertilization (IVF) with donor eggs (which includes the donor's fee and medications) in the New York City area has been estimated at $20,000, with a success rate of about 50% and some patients undergoing as many as three IVF cycles to become parents [Mead 1999]. These costs have raised concerns, like those raised in the context of adoption, that many infertile individuals are being priced out of the market [Mead 1999].

The fees paid to gamete donors have likewise increased, although most dramatically in the arena of egg donation as opposed to sperm donation. Payment for sperm and eggs is generally legal, as only the state of Louisiana has explicitly banned payment to gamete donors [Andrews 1998]. Just as demand for Caucasian infants to adopt has exceeded the number of infants available for adoption, the demand for eggs currently far exceeds the supply, and consequently, the cost of donated eggs has increased significantly [Lyke 1999a]. Lyke [1999a] points out that a decade ago, the average fee paid to an egg donor was $250, which even at that rate, was five times the $50 fee typically paid to sperm donors. Clinics currently pay egg donors between $1,500 and $5,000 [Lyke 1999a], fees that are considerably higher than fees paid to sperm donors and which generally are justified on the basis of the greater discomfort, inconvenience, and risk that egg donors experience.

Fees paid to egg donors by clinics, however, represent only one aspect of the market dynamics surrounding egg acquisition. Increasingly, independent searches for egg donors have been associated with escalating donor fees. Media attention, for example, recently focused on the efforts of an anonymous couple to obtain a desirable egg donor through an advertisement in school newspapers at Ivy League universities. The couple offered $50,000 to "a(n)[egg] donor who was at least 5-foot-10, athletic, healthy, with no family history of illness, and an SAT score of 1400-plus" [Lyke 1999a, p. 5]. Just as individuals may seek "adoptable" children of desirable physical and intellectual qualities and may evidence a willingness to pay more than prevailing agency fees to achieve their goal, the pursuit of desirable eggs may involve the payment of over-market fees. Fees also may be enhanced by "gifts" to donors. One egg-donor brokering program, for example, reports that its egg donors have received "some fabulous gifts," including cruises and college tuition [Mead 1999, p. 62]. Lyke [1999a, p. 5] criticizes this trend, asking "Should people with bigger bucks be able to buy better genes?" Others, however, defend the escalating fees and gratuities for eggs as simply paying "premium rates for hard-to-come-by goods" [Mead 1999, citing Pinkerton].

As Mead [1999, p. 59] notes, "the United States is the only country in the world in which the rules of the marketplace govern the trade in gametes and genes." In many European countries, most Latin American countries, and all Muslim countries, egg donation is prohibited [Mead 1999]. In some countries, fees associated with egg donation are strictly regulated, as in Britain where individuals may donate or sell eggs that are left over from their own in vitro fertilization cycles but where women may be paid only for time and inconvenience when they voluntarily "donate" their eggs [Mead 1999]. The United States is viewed by some as "something of a rogue nation" with regard to its commercialized egg-related practices [Mead 1999, p. 59].

These market forces in the U.S. environment, however, have not gone entirely without criticism. Some reproductive specialists in the United States have urged governmental intervention to place assisted reproduction within a framework that creates greater accountability, particularly with regard to the fees charged [Lyke 1999a, p. 8]. Some advocate that fees for donor gametes be limited, while others press for a prohibition on any reimbursement to anonymous donors [Lyke 1999a, p. 8]. Others oppose any regulatory effort, maintaining that developments along this line would require clinics to rely "on the kindness of strangers," a change in practice that would, in effect, "kill the program" [Lyke 1999a, p. 8].

The controversy in the United States, however, has centered less on whether to pay egg donors, and more on how much donors should be paid [Mead 1999]. Altruistic motives continue to be an expectation in egg donation even though donors are paid, and some clinics reject prospective donors whose only motivation appears to be the money they will receive [Jean Benward, personal communication, June 26, 2000; Mead 1999]. Mead [1999, p. 60] notes that this policy stems from the preferences of recipients for a donor who is performing the service "out of the goodness of her heart" [Mead 1999, p. 60]. In this vein, some criticize the increase in donor fees as an undesirable and "obvious shift away from altruism" [Lyke 1999a, p. 4]. Mead [1999, p. 60], however, remarks on the conflicting expectations of egg donors with regard to appropriate motivation, noting that women are expected, on the one hand, to be "compassionate toward an infertile stranger" but, on the other, to readily yield their "own genetic kin" for a limited fee.

Payments to Surrogates and Other Pregnant Women

The debate regarding money in assisted reproduction has extended to the issue of compensation to surrogates, which typically is in the range of $8,000 to $15,000 [Hirschman 1991; Jean Benward, personal communication, June 26, 2000]. The acceptability of paid surrogacy is hotly debated. Hirschman [1991, p. 10] observes that the substantial ethical controversy around surrogacy stems from "the commercial aspects of surrogacy technology" and "the intentional conception of a child who will be given up by its natural mother in return for money." Opposition to paid surrogacy centers on concerns that fees for surrogacy create "an underclass of breeder women, perhaps evoking visions of 1984 or Brave New World" [Holbrook 1990, p. 335]; children are commodified when they are carried by paid surrogates [Holbrook 1990]; and surrogacy "improperly undermines the practice of adoption" [Andrews 1998, p. 14-33, citing the Court of Cassation of France]. Those who support paid surrogacy argue that surrogate mothers are not paid for the baby but rather for their time and effort and the pain associated with giving birth, and when the intended father is the genetic father, payments to the surrogate mother simply constitute paternal support [Holbrook 1990]. Others support payments to surrogates on autonomy grounds, arguing that a woman has a right to do as she wishes with her own body, including renting the space in her womb [Freedberg 1989].

Similar concerns may be raised in adoption when a woman's expenses are paid during pregnancy and, at least from a legal standpoint, are not to be contingent on the relinquishment of her infant. It is legal for adoptive parents to pay birth parents' expenses for medical care and in some cases, living and travel expenses during pregnancy [Boskey & Hollinger 1998]. These laws, however, vary significantly from one state to another. Some states specifically define the expenses that may be paid [see Vermont Statutes 1999]; others broadly refer to "reasonable and necessary expenses" [see Arizona Revised Statutes 1999]; and yet others are known for their very permissive rules, such as Louisiana, where according to one writer, "laws are lax...the business is unregulated, and...adoption lawyers from across the country often come to nest" [Escobar 1998, p. C1].

Zelizer [1985, p. 204] notes that given the ambiguities around the payments of birth parents' expenses, the "boundary between a legitimate market and a 'dangerous' sale is not always easy to maintain." Wright [cited in Mansnerus 1998, p. A16] similarly observes that there is now only the thinnest line between "buying a child" and "buying adoption services that lead to a child." The concerns around these realities are heightened by the "considerable uncertainty. . . as to what constitutes an unlawful payment" and the generally weak sanctions when a payment is obviously improper [Boskey & Hollinger 1998, pp. 3-29].

Ethical Issues Regarding Payment

Payments to sperm donors, egg donors, surrogates and birth mothers raise a number of questions. These issues focus on what is being paid for, how much is paid, and to what extent payment affects decision making. First, paraphrasing Macklin [1996, p. 107], "what are individuals paid for and does it matter?" The prevailing rule appears to be that it is ethically permissible to pay for individuals' services (for the production of their gametes or surrogacy services) or pay the expenses incurred by prospective birth mothers in the course of pregnancy, but it is not ethically acceptable to pay for body parts or for children. Can it be determined with any fair degree of certainty whether someone is paid for a gamete or a baby as opposed to their time, inconvenience, and risk (in assisted reproduction) or reasonable living expenses (in adoption)? Does the possibility that it is the egg, the sperm, or the baby that is being purchased make an ethical difference?

A second issue relates to the level of payment and whether, ethically, there should be limits on the amount that is paid. In this context, the assumption is that payments to donors and birth parents in and of themselves are ethically permissible, but that the level of payment may need to be limited in some way. Much of this debate centers on issues of commercialization or commodification as escalating amounts of money are paid in adoption and assisted reproduction, an issue that will be discussed in greater detail later. In the arena of assisted reproduction, the debate regarding level of payment has been most intense in the context of egg donation [Macklin 1996; Mead 1999]. Some experts strongly support high fees to egg donors because of the risks involved in the procedure given the invasiveness of egg extraction [Lyke 1999b] and the uncertainties regarding the long-term effect of egg donation, including the extent to which donation may result in ovarian scarring and compromise the woman's own fertility [Mead 1999]. Others, however, raise questions regarding the extent to which increasingly higher fees place pressures on all parties concerned "to perform in less than ethical ways" [Lyke 1999a, p. 3].

The American Society for Reproductive Medicine (ASRM) [2000] in its current guidelines, allows the reimbursement of egg donors but recommends limits on such reimbursement. The guidelines allow donors to be paid the "direct and indirect expenses associated with their participation," and to be compensated for "their inconvenience, time, discomfort, and for the risk undertaken," and further provide that payments to egg donors "should not be so excessive as to constitute coercion or exploitation" [ASRM 2000, p. 10]. These guidelines compare in some ways to legal standards in adoption related to payments to pregnant women for "reasonable expenses" during pregnancy when they are contemplating adoption, payments that must be reported to courts that finalize adoptions. The nature of the guidelines as recommendations as opposed to law and the absence of any judicial or other oversights, however, limit the extent to which they may exert significant control on practice.

The third issue related to money is the extent to which payment (in assisted reproduction) or reimbursement (in adoption) works in favor of or against voluntary decision-making by donors, surrogates, and birth parents. As Macklin [1996, p. 111] notes, "the more voluntariness...can be questioned, the more ethically worrisome it is." High fees raise the possibility that the autonomy of donors, who typically are less economically advantaged than recipients, may be compromised by the financial component of the donation and relinquishment process [see Harris 1992]. This concern highlights the undue influence that high payment levels may exert on those who possess what more powerful parties (recipients, prospective adoptive parents, and service providers) desire.

Braverman [1999] writes that egg donors may bear a higher psychological risk when they donate out of need rather than choice, providing eggs for more affluent women due to economic disadvantage. Little research, however, has been conducted on the education, occupational backgrounds, or socioeconomic status of egg donors, or the effects of donation on donor women whose decisions flow from economic necessity. Some attention has been given in both domestic and international adoption to issues related to poor women placing their children for adoption with affluent (and often Caucasian) families, and this body of work may help to frame issues that may similarly arise in assisted reproduction. It is clear that socioeconomic status has played a powerful role in adoption [Howe 1995, 1997; Perry 1998]. Mandell [1973], for example, writes that adoption has been based on and has reinforced class inequities in which the affluent, as a group, historically have dominated the poor and the socially stigmatized, and Benet [1976, p. 70] refers to the power of "the white ruling group" in regulating the reproductive behavior of poor women. Research suggests, in line with concerns about the powerlessness of women with limited resources, that many women who place their infants for adoption in the United States do so because they cannot afford to raise their children themselves and this dynamic has a powerful effect on birth mothers' subsequent life experiences [Edwards 1999]. It is not clear whether issues related to socioeconomic disparity arise in assisted reproduction and, if so, what effect decision-making based on financial need will later have on donors. Much more needs to be understood regarding the socioeconomic backgrounds and needs of donors, as compared to birth parents, and the extent to which economic issues play a role in decision-making in egg donation and affect longer-term outcomes for donors.

The Role of Marketing

Personal and professional advertising has become a fixture in adoption and assisted reproduction [Gritter 1999b; Macklin & White 1997]. The use of marketing itself and the form that such marketing takes has led to a number of questions with ethical implications in both areas.

Marketing in Adoption

Personal and professional advertising are widespread in adoption. Personal advertising is typically used by prospective adoptive parents seeking pregnant women who may be considering adoption for their infants. Personal advertisements are placed in national newspapers such as USA Today and college newspapers and appear on the Internet. Typically, prospective adoptive parents highlight their financial ability to provide extremely well for a child whom they wish to adopt, including descriptions of their homes and their ability to provide exciting family vacations and enriched life experiences for a child. Gritter [1999b, p. 9] maintains that such personal advertising, which he views as a cornerstone of the commercial approach to adoption, positions prospective adoptive parents as "products in need of clever packaging." Mansnerus [1998, p. A1] observes that personal advertising of this nature reflects efforts to comply with "the first commandment for couples wanting to adopt babies: Put yourselves across."

Personal advertising by prospective adoptive parents raises a number of issues. Should individuals who wish to adopt have to "market" themselves in a public arena—to essentially "sell" themselves as a quality parenting product? Is marketing of one's qualifications to be a good adoptive parent essentially the same as or radically different than marketing one's professional or vocational skills? Should relationships leading to the adoptive placement of a child be instigated through the medium of advertising? [Freundlich 2000]. Finally, does such personal advertising have a tarnishing effect on the public perception of adoption? Does advertising, as Gritter [1999b, p. 10] suggests, portray adoption not as a "well-reasoned, well-organized institution" but as "a mad scramble of desperate families clamoring for attention"?

In addition to personal advertising by prospective adoptive parents, adoption agencies and adoption attorneys extensively advertise their services. Both groups of professionals utilize marketing techniques to recruit adoptive parents and prospective birth parents. A recent review of advertising by adoption professionals in a leading adoption magazine [Freundlich 2000] found that agencies tend to focus their efforts on attracting prospective adoptive parents, with particular emphasis on international adoption opportunities. Advertising commonly utilizes pictures of children (often swathed in lace, ribbons, or designer fabrics or sporting cowboy hats or ethnic attire) and sometimes contains descriptive titles such as "Romanian princesses," "China dolls," and "Vietnamese beauties." Agency logos vary, but were found to include, as one example, the continent of Africa over which was interposed a large eye from which a tear dropped (by an agency that arranged for adoptions of African children), and, as another example, a stork in flight with a heart-shaped object dangling from its beak (by an agency that highlights its specialization in "Caucasian newborns"). Although some agencies use tag lines that focus on children ("Making a better life for children since 1972"; "Every child deserves a loving family"; "Thousands of orphans need loving families—can you help just one?"), others attempt to respond to adult frustrations and desires ("Are you still waiting?" "Why are you still waiting?" "Realize your dreams in nine months." "This could be YOU!"). Attorney advertising in magazines tends to highlight expertise and personal status ("Proud adoptive parent"), and, unlike advertising by adoption agencies, typically offers a range of options that includes both adoption and surrogacy services. In some cases, attorneys attempt to promote their services through comforting messages, such as that of one attorney on the Internet, at the website www.youcanadopt.com, who assures prospective parents, *"I really care."*

A review of advertising approaches that target birth parents indicates a greater concentration of adoption agency marketing in the yellow pages of telephone directories than in adoption magazines. A review of the New York City Yellow Pages conducted in the spring of 2000 revealed a mixture of messages targeted to birth parents, ranging from attempts to respond to the crisis nature of unplanned pregnancy ("Confused? Pregnant? Don't Panic" and "Help is a Phone Call Away") to efforts to communicate greater empowerment for birth parents ("Open Adoption—You Choose Your Baby's Parents") to simple descriptions of services ("Choices and Services for Pregnant Women"). Lawyers, more so than adoption agencies, appear to utilize newspapers and Internet sites in an attempt to reach birth parents. One lawyer, for example, provides birth parents who happen upon her advertisement in USA Today [1999, p.10D] with a glowing description of the benefits that her clients (prospective adoptive parents) could provide to a child: "Storytelling/giggle sharing, cookie baker, t-ball, pony rides, YES!!"

Finally, there is the advertising of adoption facilitators who function in much the same way as brokers in assisted reproduction, as discussed later. As an example, one facilitator, at www.adoptlink.com, utilizes the Internet to post newborns by race and gender, displaying this and other information on a grid that displays the babies (identified by pseudonyms) whose birth dates fall within six months. The various columns of the grid indicate the child's race; gender, if known; the mother's prenatal health status; and the fees for the adoption. The fees vary, with the highest fees associated with the adoption of children identified as "white"; intermediate range fees for the adoption of children whose backgrounds are described as "one-half white and one-half African American"; and the lowest fees for the adoption of children whose backgrounds are described, for example, as "one-eighth white, one-eighth Korean, one-fourth African American, and one-half Guianese."

The advertising of adoption agencies and attorneys raises a number of issues. To what extent does such marketing play on the emotions of prospective adoptive parents and of prospective birth parents? Is it appropriate to use advertising techniques in adoption that may be effective in other product-oriented businesses— engaging photographs, catchy tag lines, bold logos, and promises of quick or economical results? And, importantly, does advertising, either in whole or in part, reflect a commodification of children? [Freundlich 2000].

Marketing in Assisted Reproduction

Personal advertising in assisted reproduction typically is utilized by prospective recipients seeking egg donors. Like prospective adoptive parents, infertile couples may advertise in college newspapers and the Internet to recruit a desired egg donor, often in conjunction with considerably higher offers than the fees paid by clinics [Lyke 1999a, p. 6]. As opposed to the more independent use of advertising by prospective recipients, donors typically use the services of brokers in advertising the availability of their eggs. Lyke [1999a, p. 4] notes:

> Dozens of brokerages have sprung up on the Internet, with fetching photos of young [egg] donor wannabes, accompanied by profiles discussing their education, grade-point averages, height, weight, personality traits, hobbies, talents and favorite movies and books.

In addition, a growing number of Internet sites, which may or may not be sponsored by egg donor programs, provide opportunities for both donors and recipients to post advertisements. Describing these posted ads as, by turns, both "poignant and outlandish," Mead [1999, p. 59] offers as one example a donor's posting that read, "I donated to a famous couple, WHY NOT YOU?" Many such sites include personal profiles, pictures, and medical histories of prospective donors (see, for example, www.eggdonor.net) to facilitate prospective recipients' selection of desirable donor attributes [Deam 2000].

Most infamously in this regard, an Internet website entitled Ron's Angels advertised in 1999 the auction of the eggs of supermodels. Purporting to broker ultra-eggs, "Ron" stated:

> If you could increase the chance of reproducing beautiful children and thus giving them an advantage in society, would you?...This is Darwin's natural selection at its very best. The highest bidder gets youth and beauty...It is not my intention to suggest we make a super society of only beautiful people. This site simply mirrors our current society, in that beauty always goes to the highest bidder.

Although the site ultimately proved a hoax, the attention that it attracted reflected, according to Annas [1999], the general belief that anything can be sold to the highest bidder, including beauty. Goldberg [1999] observes that the website's "melding of Darwin-based eugenics, Playboy-style sensibilities and eBay-type commerce" represents "the most worrying sign yet of where the partly unregulated field of assisted reproduction may be going."

Marketing by assisted reproduction service providers also has increased significantly. Macklin and White [1997, p. 128] note that assisted reproduction "has become a prime target for the marketing and advertising techniques common in American culture." Some commentators point to the "ingenious" marketing strategies of egg-donation programs, in particular [Mead 1999, p. 58]. Mead [1999, pp. 58-59], for example, describes the following marketing techniques:

A New York egg-donation program advertises in movie theaters, inviting would-be donors to dial 1-877-BABY MAKERS. A new company in Los Angeles called the Center for Egg Options hired a hip advertising agency to write catchy ad copy. Instead of variations on the usual "give the gift of life" theme, one ad reads simply, "Pay your tuition with eggs." Another...says, "Get paid $4,000 for a small part." The same company is known for sending fertility doctors promotional giveaways that consist of shrink-wrapped egg cartons filled with chocolate eggs.

There are conflicting views of the propriety of advertising in assisted reproduction. Some believe that "advertising is not in and of itself devoid of ethics but perhaps inadequate for the task of maintaining the status and dignity of human reproduction" [Macklin & White 1997, p. 128]. Others favor "practical but non-regulatory routes for pursuing fairness in marketing practices and accuracy in advertising," an issue that has been raised less in relation to the marketing strategies that are used and more in connection with clinics' advertising regarding their "success" rates [Macklin & White 1997, p. 128].

The provision of accurate and clear information on programs' success in terms of the number of live births achieved (characterized as one of the "most intractable goals to accomplish" [Macklin & White 1997, p. 128]) raises key ethical issues in the context of much of the advertising by assisted reproduction service providers. The debate has centered principally on the nature of the information that is conveyed to prospective patients in promoting the benefits of individual programs. Some believe that ethically, clinics should publicize only their actual birth rates so that consumers are informed of the "true" success rates achieved; others contend that publicizing expected, as opposed to actual, birth rates is ethically acceptable as such information can provide timely and useful guidance to the consumer [Macklin & White 1997]. The nuances of this debate are beyond the scope of this paper, but the issues are important in evaluating the nature of advertising in an environment in which, like adoption, consumers may be eager, if not desperate, for the promise of success.

Children and Offspring as Product

The question of commercialization, if not commodification, arises in both adoption and assisted reproduction. Just as increasing fees in adoption (particularly for racially desirable and healthy infants) have precipitated concerns related to commodification of children [Gritter 1999b; Watson 1999], higher fees to donors in assisted reproduction have been criticized as contributing to the commodification of gametes and to the transformation of babies into products that doctors manufacture [Mead 1999].

In adoption, the increasing role of money has raised the issue of whether infants have been transformed into commodities rated on certain characteristics, with the most desirable children (healthy, Caucasian infants) available to those individuals who are able to pay the highest fee [Freundlich 2000]. These concerns raise a number of questions. Are infants simply another product that may be purchased by those who are able and willing to pay the most money? Has money essentially changed the nature of infant adoption from a service for children to a service for affluent adults?

In assisted reproduction, the issue of commodification arises in several contexts, posing the question whether, as Hirschman [1991, p. 4] notes, it is children "who are for sale." Payments to surrogates, for example, are viewed by some as reflecting a consumer product orientation because the children's very existence is:

> prenegotiated, predesigned, and contracted for just like any other commercial transaction. The child is a product with his or her status indistinguishable from other manufactured goods. [Holbrook 1990, p. 335].

Similarly, others point to the indirect commodification of children through a view of eggs as products and a view of donors as suppliers. Recipients may have specific expectations regarding the characteristics of donors (and, by extension, their eggs) much in the same way that prospective adoptive parents may have expectations regarding birth parents and the children they will adopt. Mead [1999, p. 62] notes that recipients "expect to be offered donors who are not just healthy but bright, accomplished, and attractive." She [1999, p. 62] suggests that commercialization lies at the basis of this expectation:

> Egg donor recipients bridle at the suggestion that they are shopping for genes, but the agencies and the programs provide so much personal information about donors that recipients are invited to view eggs as merchandise.

The market for sperm, eggs, and embryos has been described as "in a state of disarray," marked by a perplexing combination of altruism and commercialization [Hirschman 1991, p. 18]. Sperm, eggs, and embryos may be provided altruistically, but, unlike blood, kidneys, and other organs that may not be purchased, they are for sale [Hirschman 1991]. Hirschman [1991, p. 4] notes that this inconsistency in the ethics of acquisition of human body parts "has received little attention in consumer policy literature, yet is growing rapidly in monetary size and societal significance." Is Hirschman [1991, p. 5] correct in suggesting that assisted reproduction, from a market perspective, is "centered around the production and acquisition of babies"? Or, is the act of commercialization not necessarily a negative feature of the market because, as Hough [1978] suggests, it rectifies the imbalance between supply and demand? Or, is it more appropriate to distinguish sperm, egg, and embryo donations based on what is being purchased? Berg [1995, p. 88], for example, writes:

> While egg donors are paid irrespective of whether or not pregnancy results—that is, they are paid for the egg extraction process, [for] sperm donors...compensation appears to be provided more for the sperm itself, rather than for the process of providing the sperm. Similarly, compensation in contract motherhood arrangements, which is ostensibly for the services of gestation and childbirth, is not provided if the child is not turned over

to the infertile couple. Therefore, the payment appears to be for the child and not for the process of gestation. Only oocyte donation appears to circumvent the symbolic purchase of a child or of life-giving potential.

The potential for commodification of children through a "gametes as merchandise" paradigm is an issue that is far from resolution. Clearly, one aspect of paid "donation" that requires more attention is its meaning for the child born from such an arrangement [Mead 1999]. One commentator notes that "no one considers how the child feels when she finds that her natural father was a $25 cup of sperm" [Rubin 1983]. Alternatively, how will a resulting child view the $50,000 purchase of the ideal egg that led to her conception? These issues, to some extent, have surfaced in adoption when adoptees learn that they were adopted in exchange for a great sum of money [Gritter 1999b]. One attorney known for his work in arranging independent adoptions has argued that the impact can only be positive:

> How would I feel if my father paid ten thousand dollars to adopt me? Boy, that guy really wanted me...He paid that much for me, he really wanted me that much...What could be a greater sense of self than that somebody sacrificed so much to have me?...[McTaggart 1980, p. 318, quoting Stanley Michelman].

Child welfare professionals typically express skepticism of this rationale for charging large fees, particularly as it seems to suggest that the higher the fee the better, an outcome of none-too-incidental benefit to the very adoption professionals who advance this line of reasoning. Gritter [1999b, p. 11], for example, writes, "For the child, there is no consolation for the thought that one has been sold and purchased."

The issues of commercialization and commodification raise important issues. Macklin [1996, p. 120] remarks that commodification may not be "immoral," but:

> It is nonetheless unsavory. This category of disvalue does not involve a violation of ethical principle; yet it rests on

the conviction that not every human exchange ought to be subject to market forces.

The extent to which these market forces should be allowed to operate raises key questions about who is accountable to whom in assisted reproduction, an ethical question of equal concern in adoption.

Chapter 6

Embryo Donation and Adoption

The concept of embryo donation—or "embryo adoption" as it is sometimes described—raises some unique issues. Embryo donation can occur in two ways: an individual may receive a preexisting cryopreserved embryo or an embryo may be specifically created with donated eggs and donated sperm [Cooper & Glazer 1998]. In the first situation, a couple donates the stored embryos they produced but did not use in an earlier in vitro fertilization (IVF) procedure [Rubin 1998]. Some assert that the demand for the preserved embryos of others has grown substantially and that even individuals who could use their own eggs and sperm for IVF may opt for donor embryos [Rubin 1998]. Jean Benward [personal communication, June 26, 2000], however, points out that the practice of embryo donation has remained largely unidentified, and few reports on the prevalence of embryo donation have been published.

In one of the few studies on the issue, the American Society of Reproductive Medicine (ASRM) Mental Health Professional Group found that in 1996, 72% of the IVF programs in the United States that responded to its survey claimed that they offered embryo donation to patients, but only 37% actually performed embryo donation, reporting 53 babies born from the process [Kingsberg et al. 2000]. Jean Benward[personal communication June 26, 2000] suggests that these survey results reflect that although thousands of frozen embryos remain in cryopreservation, embryo donation has been relatively uncommon thus far. She further notes, however, that since the ASRM survey, some IVF programs have begun to advertise embryo adoption services. Rubin [1998] similarly notes the increased advertising related to embryo adoption, particularly the lower cost of the service (in the range of $5,000) compared to significantly greater sums for an IVF cycle and even higher fees if a donor egg is used [Rubin 1998].

In addition to embryo adoption, some clinics have begun to offer a second process, "embryo creation," in which male and female donor gametes are utilized to create embryos specifically for the purpose of a transfer [Cooper & Glazer 1998]. Cooper and Glazer [1998, p. 3] write that "although both methods result in an offspring who is not genetically connected to the parents, from an ethical, emotional, and social policy perspective, these two avenues to embryo adoption are decidedly different." One view of embryo creation is that it is simply "a logical extension of single gamete donation" [Kolata 1997]; the other view is that it is a "supermarket approach" [Kolata 1997] that is "tantamount to creating children for adoption" [Cooper & Glazer 1998, p. 2].

It is not clear to what extent "embryo creation" may be utilized as some clinics have refused to engage in the practice [Jean Benward, personal communication, June 26, 2000]. Nonetheless, criticisms of "embryo creation" raise important issues with implications for both adoption and assisted reproduction in general. The criticisms of "embryo creation" center on the perception that adults are seeking higher levels of control over the "design" of their children and that the process offers greater benefits in this regard than is possible when an existing embryo is selected [Cooper & Glazer 1998, p. 2].

Prospective parents' control over the characteristics of the child whom they will parent has become a key issue in relation to adoption and assisted reproduction, with the level of control clearly varying across the array of available parenting options. Adopting an existing child provides adults with no control over the child's genetic makeup, and information on birth family genetic history is generally limited to birth parent reports (with, often, the birth father's information being quite limited); the "adoption" of a preexisting embryo does not provide control over the future child's genetic makeup but gives intended parents somewhat greater access to information on the genetics of the donors of egg and sperm (although practice varies, as discussed previously); and "embryo creation" provides adults with a significant level of control over the future child's genetic makeup as they can select egg and sperm donors and optimize the probabilities of desired characteristics. Should adults be given the opportunity to "design" their children in ways that match their parenting interests and needs? Are efforts along this line simply a proxy for the genetic control inherent in biological procreation? Or, do such efforts represent a consumer orientation that extends to "designer" children? What does "design control" suggest about the children who are subsequently created? How do existing children in need of families fit into such a paradigm?

It appears that for many individuals, embryo donation is preferable to adoption for reasons other than the opportunity to have greater control over the genetic makeup of the child. For many infertile individuals, embryo adoption can provide the desired experience of pregnancy and prenatal bonding. The process further provides the recipient with the opportunity to regulate the prenatal environment, completely if she carries the embryo herself and partially if she selects a surrogate. This opportunity contrasts with traditional adoption in which the prospective parents may not know the birth mother until later in the pregnancy or not at all, and, thus, may have only limited information on the mother's prenatal health status and her medical care. Further, health, genetic, and other information on egg and sperm donors may exceed the information typically available on birth parents in a traditional adoption. Pragmatically, embryo adoption may be far more affordable than traditional adoption given the fees typically involved, and it is likely to involve far less legal and other paper work [Embryo Adoption 1999]. Finally, "traditional adoption, by definition, is always public, whereas embryo adoption can be private, allowing the couple to reveal it when and to whom they choose" [Cooper & Glazer 1998, p. 2].

The similarities and differences between so-called traditional adoption and embryo adoption have not been fully explored. One adoption agency, (the Snowflake Embryo Adoption Program), however, has initiated what is "believed to be the first adoption service designed to unite childless couples with the fertilized eggs from previous infertility treatments" [Richardson 1999, p. 1].

Contending that the process is not merely the donation of an embryo but an adoption, the program treats frozen embryos as the equivalent of full-fledged, parentless children who need to be rescued from their "frozen orphanages" [Richardson 1999, p. 3]. Viewing embryos as requiring the same protection as children in need of adoptive placements, the agency requires couples petitioning for an embryo to be screened to determine whether they are fit to parent and advocates for "laws requiring prospective parents to undergo background checks, home visits and other adoption requirements before receiving embryos for implantation" [Richardson 1999, p. 3].

The view that prospective recipients of donated embryos are the equivalent of prospective adoptive parents of existing children raises a number of questions. Should the practice of embryo donation be subject to the rules governing adoption? Does the extension of adoption principles to embryo donation suggest that children and embryos are the same and have equivalent interests? Is there a sufficiently solid base in adoption to extend its assessment processes related to parental fitness to assisted reproduction?

Many of the complexities associated with articulating the principles that should guide embryo adoption flow from the dilemma of defining embryos either as people or property [Andrews 1999]. At the policy level, there is considerable reluctance to define an embryo in definitive terms as either. The Waller Committee of Australia in 1984, for example, recommended that an "embryo should not be afforded the status of 'personhood' (but)...it merits more respect than an entity created solely for research purposes" [cited in Cucci 1998, p. 421]. Similarly, the Warnock Committee in the United Kingdom declared that "the human embryo...is not, under the present law in the UK, accorded the same status as a living child or an adult," although it recommended that the embryo be given a "special status" [cited in Cucci 1998, p. 421]. In 1979, the Ethics Advisory Board of the U.S. Department of Health, Education, and Welfare issued a statement calling for the respect of the human embryo because of its "potential to become a person" but, nonetheless, declared that an embryo did not warrant the full legal and moral rights of a human being [cited in Cucci 1998, p. 422]. In 1984, the Ethics Committee of the American Fertility Society similarly concluded that "the [embryo] is due greater respect than any other human tissue because of its potential to become a person...Yet, it should not be treated as a person, because it has not yet developed the features of personhood, is not yet established as developmentally individual, and may never realize its biologic potential" [cited in Cucci 1998, p. 422].

The courts, however, by necessity, have reached more definite conclusions regarding the status of embryos. In one Tennessee case, a court ruled that the seven frozen embryos of a couple in the process of divorce were not property, but, in fact, were "children" with "a right to be born" [cited in Andrews 1999]. The court of appeals, however, reversed that decision, rejecting the characterization of embryos as persons with legal and moral rights [Mahoney 1995]. A Virginia court explicitly relied on property principles in a case involving a patient whose Virginia clinic had denied her request for the transfer of her embryos to a doctor in another state [Andrews 1999]. As Mahoney [1995, p. 41] points out, courts, when asked to distinguish the status of embryos as property or as children, face significant challenges "perhaps because (embryos) are neither."

Both the principles of embryos as "property" and as "people" present issues with significant implications for practice. Andrews [1999] contends that "what the property analogy clearly does is to accentuate the trend to view the children of reproductive technology as consumer goods" and to give legitimacy to couples who wish to "order" the traits of their future children as they would any other consumer good. "As sperm, eggs and embryos are treated more and more like consumer products, people's expectations increase about the resulting children—and the law is called in when they are disappointed" [Andrews 1999]. Characterizing embryos as "people" also raises a host of issues. If an embryo is considered a human being, it presumably would be entitled "to all the rights of personhood...with a duty to protect...embryos from harm" [Cucci 1998, p. 422]. As "people," embryos, having been purposefully created, would presumably have a right not to be discarded by either the genetic contributors or the clinic at which they are housed. These principles have been statutorily recognized to some degree in Louisiana legislation that recognizes human embryos as "juridical person(s) which may not be intentionally destroyed, and which hold even at the one-call stage, the right to sue or be sued through an appointed curator" [cited in Cucci 1998, p. 423]. The "person" approach to embryos may avert the commodification issue that Andrews [1999] identifies in relation to the "embryos as property" paradigm, but it raises other issues. Are embryos, as "persons," equivalent to existing children in need of adoptive families? Should there be a "best interest" or other standard to guide services to embryos? Would the existence of "personhood" entitle an embryo to adoption if the genetic contributors do not wish to utilize the embryo for a pregnancy?

Chapter 7

The Law of Adoption and Assisted Reproduction

Although the parent-child relationship resulting from assisted reproduction parallels adoption because children are added to families with whom they have a partial or no genetic connection, the nature and level of regulation of the two areas differ significantly. Because adoption is the more established form of non-traditional family formation, the law more comprehensively addresses the nature of parent-child relationships [Hollinger 1999a]. Adoption occurs within a legal and regulatory structure and, to a greater or lesser degree, oversight mechanisms are in place. Agencies must be licensed; adoption attorneys must be members of bar associations that oversee professional practice; and courts must finalize adoptions. It should be noted, however, that the laws vary widely from state to state and although some aspects of adoption are well regulated (the requirement that adoptive parents have approved home studies, for example, and clear definitions of the rights of adoptive parents), other aspects of the practice may be subject to varying degrees of oversight, including the fees and expenses charged [Hollinger 1999a].

The variability in adoption law aside, however, the extent to which the law regulates adoption clearly far exceeds the regulation of assisted reproduction. Andrews [1999, p. 3] notes that although "there are pages of adoption laws on the books in each state, only three states—Florida, Virginia and New Hampshire—have enacted legislation to address reproductive technology in any comprehensive fashion" [Andrews 1999, p. 3]. Instead, the law of assisted reproduction has evolved slowly through case law and issue-specific statutory provisions that are reactive to emerging issues. The advent of artificial insemination, for example, precipitated the need to define legal fatherhood outside of biology or adoption. Faced with determining paternity when a wife had been inseminated by donor sperm, courts opted to hold the woman's husband as the legal father, viewing his consent to insemination as "an alternative to following traditional adoption procedure" [Andrews 1998, pp. 14-6, 14-7]. Current statutes have continued this approach, and a husband who consents to donor insemination holds the status of legal father and the sperm donor holds no rights to or responsibilities for the child [Andrews 1998].

The law, however, is less clear regarding determinations of parenthood when egg donation and embryo donation are involved. A few states have enacted legislation that specifies that donors have no legal responsibility for children who are conceived through the donation of their eggs (an approach that is consistent with laws related to the obligations of sperm donors), but most states have not addressed this issue [Mead 1999]. Andrews [1998, p. 14-10] speculates that in states where such statutes are not in place, "it is likely that courts will view the situation as analogous to sperm donation and find that adoption laws do not apply." If this approach proves to be correct, the woman who is the egg recipient would, by virtue of her consent, be the legal mother when she carries an embryo created with a donated egg and her husband's sperm. It is not clear, however, that parenthood would automatically vest if the woman carried an embryo to which neither she nor her husband had contributed genetically. In such cases, would the fact of gestational mothering suffice to confer legal parent status? Or, would adoption law be more applicable?

As discussed earlier, courts' rulings in surrogacy generally have focused on genetic relationships and/or the intent to parent. In traditional surrogacy cases (in which the father has contributed sperm and the intended mother has no genetic connection with the child), however, the intended mother typically has been required to adopt the child [Andrews 1998]. Andrews [1998, p. 14-10] notes that this area of assisted reproduction is "where the strongest argument can be made for application of some of the other aspects of the adoption model." Should the same analysis apply to gestational surrogacy cases and both the intended father and intended mother be required to adopt?

Agreement appears to exist that there is a need for a more fully developed legal framework that outlines the legal rights and responsibilities of parties to assisted reproduction [Andrews 1998]. The reluctance to apply adoption law in all but very limited circumstances raises a number of questions. Are there aspects of the adoption model that could be utilized to address some of the thorny questions related to parenthood in assisted reproduction? Or, are the differences between the two forms of family formation so distinct as to render adoption an irrelevant analogy and to require an entirely new legal approach?

Chapter 8

Conclusion

The adoption of infants and assisted reproduction involving donor gametes share a number of characteristics [see Benward 2000]:

- A common originating point in infertility;

- The involvement of multiple parties in family formation;

- The lack of genetic connectedness between at least one parent and child;

- The social stigma that may be associated with both services as nontraditional means of forming a family;

- A history of treating information as confidential that extends to the parties to the services themselves;

- The role of professionals in "managing" the process of family formation; and

- Aspects of the "business" of each service that potentially impact the essential function of each service.

At the same time, there are key differences between infant adoption and assisted reproduction with donor gametes [see Benward 2000]:

- Differences in the nature of the relationships created through each service, with greater complexity in assisted reproduction by virtue of genetic, gestational, and social factors;

- Different roles for the parties who make the respective services possible (birth parents in adoption and donors in assisted reproduction);

- Differing perspectives on the appropriateness of greater openness among the parties to the services and the sharing of information;

- Differing social environments and differing levels of supports for the disclosure of the use of each service— to others and to the child;

- Differing service environments—a social service orientation in adoption and a medical orientation in assisted reproduction—with different implications regarding who is the "client";

- Different views of the role of the professional in the service, with greater gatekeeping responsibilities assumed by adoption professionals;

- Differing levels of regulation and oversight of the provision of services; and

- Distinctions in the extent to which the legal rights of genetic/birth parents and social/intended parents have been clearly defined.

This volume has attempted to identify some of key ethical issues that confront the fields of adoption and assisted reproduction, including the roles of the various parties to those services and how those perceived roles impact service delivery; issues bearing on anonymity and information sharing; and concerns related to the growing power of market forces in each service area. There has been some research regarding the impact of adoption on which professionals may draw in an attempt to resolve these questions. By contrast, the limited research in assisted reproduction has made it difficult to determine the relative risks and benefits of a number of aspects of current practice [Berg 1995]. Identification of the key issues, as has been attempted here, hopefully will serve as a first step toward full discussion of the challenges and resolution of the issues that professionals in adoption and assisted reproduction confront in practice and policy.

References

Abbey, A., Andrews, F. M., & Halman, L. J. (1992). Infertility and subjective well-being: The mediating roles of self-esteem, internal control, and interpersonal conflict. *Journal of Marriage and the Family, 54*(2), 408–417.

American Society for Reproductive Medicine. (2000). *Guidelines for gamete and embryo donation. A Practice Committee report.* [On-line]. Available: http://www.asrm.com/Media/Practice/gamete.html#Guidelines.

Amuzu, B., Laxova, R., & Shapiro, S. S. (1990). Pregnancy outcome, health of children, and family adjustment after donor insemination. *Obstetrics & Gynecology, 75*, 899–905.

Anderson, K. (1989). Infertility: The silent crisis. *Canada's Mental Health, 37*(1), 9–12.

Andrews, L. B. (1998). Alternative reproduction and the law of adoption. In J. H. Hollinger (Ed.), *Adoption Law and Practice, Vol. II* (pp. 14-1 to 14-43). New York: Matthew Bender.

Andrews, L. B. (1999, May 2). Embryonic confusion: When you think conception, you don't think product liability. Think again. *The Washington Post*, p. B01.

Annas, G. J. (1986). The baby broker boom. *Hastings Center Report, 16*(3), 30–31.

Annas, G. J. (1988). Death without dignity for commercial surrogacy: The case of Baby M. *Hastings Center Report, 18*(2), 21–24.

Annas, G. J. (1999, November 3). *Ethics in a world ruled by law and the market: Adoption, assisted reproduction and parenthood.* Presentation at the conference, Ethics and Adoption: Challenges for Today and the Future, Anaheim, CA (Convened by the Evan B. Donaldson Adoption Institute).

Arizona Revised Statutes. (1999). Title 8: Children. [On-line]. Available: http://www.azleg.state.az.us.

Arneson, R. J. (1992). Commodification and commercial surrogacy. *Philosophy & Public Affairs, 21*(2), 132–164.

Asche, A. (1985). *Creating children: Report of the Family Law Council of Australia.* Canberra: Australia Government Publishing Service.

Auth, P. J. & Zaret, S. (1986). The search in adoption: A service and a process. *Social Casework, 67*(9), 560–68.

Avery, R. (1996). *Information disclosure and openness in adoption: State policy and empirical evidence.* Ithaca, NY: Cornell University.

Baran, A. & Pannor, R. (1989). *Lethal secrets: The psychology of donor insemination.* New York: Amistad Press.

Barker, S., Byrne, S., Morrison, M., & Spenser, M. (1998). *Preparing for permanence. Assessment: Points to consider for those assessing potential adopters and foster carers.* London: British Agencies for Adoption and Fostering.

Bartholet, E. (1993, July 13). Op-Ed: Blood parents vs. real parents. *The New York Times*, p. A19.

Bartholet, E. (1998). Private race preferences in family formation. *Yale Law Journal, 107*(7), 2351–2356.

Benet, M. K. (1976). *The politics of adoption.* New York: Free Press.

Benward, J. (1998). Donor registries in reproductive medicine, Presentation at the 31st annual postgraduate course, *Advanced Counseling Issues: Third Party Reproduction*, San Francisco, CA (Convened by the American Society for Reproductive Medicine).

Benward, J. (2000, May 5). Creating families in third party reproduction and adoption. Chart presented at *Bridging the Gap: Adoption and Assisted Reproduction*, Chicago, IL (Convened by the Center for Clinical Medical Ethics, University of Chicago).

Benward, J. & Asch, A. (1999, November 5). *A case for cross-fertilization: Adoption and the reproductive technologies*, Presentation at the conference, Ethics and Adoption: Challenges for Today and the Future, Anaheim, CA (Convened by the Evan B. Donaldson Adoption Institute).

Berg, B. F. (1995). Listening to the voices of the infertile. In J. C. Callahan (Ed.), *Reproduction, ethics, and the law* (pp. 80–108). Indianapolis: Indiana University Press.

Berry, M., Barth, R. P., & Needell, B. (1996). Preparation, support and satisfaction of adoptive families in agency and independent adoptions. *Child and Adolescent Social Work Journal, 13*(2), 157–183.

Bezanson, R. P. (1990). Solomon would weep: A Comment on *In the Matter of Baby M* and the limits of judicial authority. In L. Gostin (Ed.), *Surrogate Motherhood: Politics and Privacy* (pp. 243–252). Indianapolis: Indiana University Press.

Black, R. B., Walther, V. N., Chute, D., & Greenfeld, D. A. (1992). When in vitro fertilization fails: A prospective view. *Social Work in Health Care, 17*(3), 1–19.

Blyth, E. (1999). Secrets and lies: Barriers to the exchange of genetic origins information following donor assisted conception. *Adoption & Fostering, 23*(1), 49–58.

Boskey, J. B. & Hollinger, J. H. (1998). Placing children for adoption. In J. H. Hollinger (Ed.), *Adoption Law and Practice* (pp. 3-1 to 3-65). New York: Matthew Bender.

Bouchier, P., Lambert, L., & Triseliotis, J. (1991). *Parting with a child for adoption: The mother's perspective.* London: British Association of Adoption and Fostering.

Braverman, A. (1993). Survey results of the current practice of ovum donation. *Fertility and Sterility, 59,* 1216–1220.

Braverman, A. (1999, Spring). Psychological issues involved in egg donation: Part 2. *Resolve National Newsletter,* pp. 6–8.

Bringhenti, F., Martinelli, F., Ardenti, R., & La Sala, G.B. (1997). Psychological adjustment of infertile women entering IVF treatment: Differentiating aspects and influencing factors. *Acta Obstetricia et Gynecologica Scandinavica, 76*(5), 431–437.

Brodzinksy, D. M. (1987). Adjustment to adoption: A psychosocial perspective. *Clinical Psychology Review, 7,* 25–47.

Brodzinsky, D. M. (1990). A stress and coping model of adoption adjustment. In D. M. Brodzinsky & M. D. Schechter (Eds.), *The Psychology of Adoption* (pp. 3–24). New York: Oxford University Press.

Brodzinsky, D. M., Lang, R., & Smith, D. W. (1995). Parenting adopted children. In M. II. Bornstein (Ed.), *Handbook of parenting, Vol. 3: Status and social conditions of parenting* (pp. 209–232). Hillsdale, NJ: Lawrence Erlbaum.

Brodzinsky, D. M., Smith, D. W. & Brodzinsky, A. B. (1998). *Children's adjustment to adoption.* Thousand Oaks, CA: Sage Publications.

Burns, L. H. (1987). Infertility as boundary ambiguity: One theoretical perspective. *Family Process, 26*(3), 359–372.

Burns, L. H. (1990). An exploratory study of perceptions of parenting after infertility. *Family Systems Medicine, 8*(2), 177–189.

Butler, R. R. & Koraleski, S. (1990). Infertility: A crisis with no resolution. *Journal of Mental Health Counseling, 12*(2), 151–163.

Byrd, D. (1998). The case for confidential adoptions. *Public Welfare, 46*(4), 20–23.

Callahan, S. (1987). The ethical challenge of the new reproductive technology. In J. E. Monagle & D. C. Thomasma (Eds.), *Medical ethics: A guide for health care professionals* (pp. 153–158). Frederick, MD: Aspen Publishers.

Carp, E. W. (1992). The sealed adoption records controversy in historical perspective: The case of the Children's Home Society of Washington, 1895–1988. *Journal of Sociology and Social Work, 19* (2), 27–57.

Carstens, C. S. (1995). Legal, policy, and practice issues for intercountry adoptions in the United States. *Adoption and Fostering, 19*(4), 26–33.

Chasin, R. (1993). Foreword. In E. Imber-Black (Ed.), *Secrets in Families and Family Therapy* (pp. vii–ix). New York: Norton.

Chelo, E., Noci, I., Barciulli, F., Bigagli, A., Coppini, A. B., Masciandaro, C., & Romani, A. (1986). The imagined baby: The analysis of a desire. *Acta Europaea Fertilitatis, 17*(3), 213–216.

Chesler, P. (1988, May 11). Remarks at a public hearing on surrogacy conducted by the New Jersey Bioethics Commission, Newark, NJ.

Clark, I., McWilliam, E., & Phillips, R. (1998). Empowering prospective adopters. *Adoption & Fostering, 22*(2), 35–43.

Cloud, J. (1999, February 22). Tracking down Mom. *Time*, 26–30.

CNN. (2000, August 24). *California court rules sperm donors privacy rights are limited.* [On-line]. Available: http://cgi.cnn.com/2000/LAW/08/24/sperm.identity.ap.

Cohen C. (1996). Parents anonymous. In C. Cohen (Ed.), *New ways of making babies: A case of egg donation*, (pp. 88–105). Bloomington: Indiana University Press.

Collins, J. A., Bustillo, M., Visscher, R. D., & Lawrence, L. D. (1995). An estimate of the cost of in vitro fertilization services in the United States in 1995. *Fertility and Sterility, 64*, 538–545.

Condon, J. T. (1986). Psychological disability in women who relinquish a baby for adoption. *Medical Journal of Australia, 144*(3), 117–119.

Cook, R., Golombok, S., Bish, A., & Murray, C. (1994). Disclosure of donor insemination: Parental attitudes. *American Journal of Orthopsychiatry, 65*(4), 549–559.

Cooper, S. L. & Glazer, E. S. (1998). Choosing embryo adoption. In S. L. Cooper & E. S. Glazer (Ed.), *Choosing assisted reproduction: Social, emotional and ethical considerations.* Indianapolis: Perspectives Press. [On-line]. Available: http://www.perspectivespress.com/ carembryo.html [1999, Nov. 11].

Craig, T. L. (1998). Establishing the biological rights doctrine to protect unwed fathers in contested adoptions. *Florida State University Law Review, 25*, 391–438.

Crockin, S. L. (1999). Where is anonymous reproduction taking us? In R. Jansen & D. Mortimer (Eds.), *Towards reproductive certainty* (pp. 467–473). New York: Parthenon Publishing Group.

Cucci, N. L. (1998). Constitutional implications of in vitro fertilization procedures. *St. John's Law Review, 72*(2), 417–449.

Daly, K. J. (1992). Toward a formal theory of interactive resocialization: The case of adoptive parenthood. *Qualitative Sociology, 15*(4), 395–417.

Daniels, K. & Lewis, G. M. (1996). Openness of information in the use of donor gametes: Developments in New Zealand. *Journal of Reproductive and Infant Psychology, 14*, 57–68.

Daniels, K. & Taylor, K. (1993, August). Secrecy and openness in donor insemination. *Politics and Life Sciences*, 155–170.

Department of Health and Social Security. (1984). *The Warnock report: Report of the Committee of Inquiry into Human Fertilisation and Embryology*, (Cmnd. 9314). London: Her Majesty's Stationary Office.

Edwards, D. S. (1995). *Transformation of motherhood in adoption: The experiences of relinquishing mothers.* Unpublished doctoral dissertation, University of North Florida, Jacksonville.

Edwards, D. S. (1999). American adoption and the experiences of relinquishing mothers. *Practicing Anthropology, 21*(1), 18–23.

Elias, S. & Annas, G. J. (1986). Noncoital reproduction. *Journal of the American Medical Association, 255*, 67.

Embryo Adoption. (1999, November 11). [On-line]. Available: http:// www.conceivingconcepts.com/embryo.htm [1999, Nov. 11].

Escobar, G. (1998, November 16). Lawyer's kidnap spotlights Louisiana adoption laws. *The Washington Post*, p. C01.

Feversham Committee. (1960). *Report of the Departmental Committee on Human Artificial Insemination*, (Cmnd. 1105). London: Her Majesty's Stationary Office.

Freedberg, S. (1989). Self-determination: Historical perspectives and effects on current practice. *Social Work, 34*(1), 33–38.

Freeman, M. (1996). The new birth right? Identity and the child of the reproduction revolution. *The International Journal of Children's Rights, 4*, 273–297.

Freundlich, M. (2000). *The market forces in adoption.* Washington, DC: Child Welfare League of America.

Freundlich, M. & Peterson, L. (1998). *Wrongful adoption: Law, policy, and practice.* Washington, DC: Child Welfare League of America.

Gill, B. (in press). Adoption agencies and the search for the ideal family, 1918–1965. In E. W. Carp (Ed.), *Adoption in history: New interpretative essays.* Lansing: University of Michigan Press.

Goldberg, C. (1999, October 23). On Web, models auction their eggs to bidders for beautiful children. *The New York Times,* p. A19.

Golombok, S. (1997). The controversy surrounding privacy or disclosure among donor gamete recipients. *Journal of Assisted Reproduction and Genetics, 14*(7), 378–80.

Golombok, S., Cook, R., Bish, A., & Murray, C. (1995). Families created by the new reproductive technologies: Quality of parenting and social and emotional development of the children. *Child Development, 66*(2), 285–298.

Golombok, S. & Murray, C. (1999). Social versus biological parenting: Family functioning and the socioemotional development of children conceived by egg or sperm donation. *Journal of Child Psychiatry, 40*, 519–527.

Goodman, K. & Rothman, B. (1984). Group work in infertility treatment. *Social Work with Groups, 7*(1), 79–97.

Gostin, L. (1990). A civil liberties analysis of surrogacy arrangements. In L. Gostin. (Ed.), *Surrogate motherhood: Politics and policy* (pp. 3–23). Bloomington, IN: Indiana University Press.

Greenfeld, D. A. (1997). Infertility and assisted reproductive technology: The role of the perinatal social worker. *Social Work in Health Care, 24*(3/4), 39–16.

Griswold v. Connecticut. (1965). 381 U.S. 479.

Gritter, J. (1999a). *The spirit of open adoption.* Washington, DC: CWLA Press.

Gritter, J. (1999b). The trend of commercialization in adoption. *Decree, 1,* 9–13.

Harris, J. (1992). *Wonderwoman and superman.* New York: Oxford University Press.

Hartman, A. & Laird, J. (1990). Family treatment after adoption: Common themes. In D. M Brodzinsky & M. D. Schechter (Eds.), *The psychology of adoption* (pp.221–239). New York: Oxford University Press.

Hirschman, E. C. (1991). Babies for sale: Market ethics and the new reproductive technologies. *Journal of Consumer Affairs, 25*(2), 358–391.

Hoffman-Riem, C. (1990). *The adopted child: Family life with double parenthood.* Piscataway, NJ: Transaction Publishers.

Holbrook, S. M. (1990). Adoption, infertility, and the new reproductive technologies: Problems and prospects for social work and welfare policy. *Social Work, 35*(4), 333–337.

Hollinger, H. F. (1985). From coitus to commerce: Legal and social consequences of noncoital reproduction. *University of Michigan Journal of Legal Reform, 18,* 891–899.

Hollinger, J. H. (1995). Adoption and aspiration: The Uniform Adoption Act, the DeBoer-Schmidt case, and the American quest for the ideal family. *Duke Journal of Gender Law & Policy, 2*(1), 15–40.

Hollinger, J. H. (1999a). Adoption procedure. In J. H. Hollinger (Ed.), *Adoption law and practice* (Vol. 1) (pp. 4-1 to 4-172). New York: Matthew Bender.

Hollinger, J. H. (1999b). Aftermath of adoption: Legal and social consequences. In J. H. Hollinger (Ed.), *Adoption law and practice* (Vol. 2) (pp. 13-1 to 13-105). New York: Matthew Bender.

Hough, D. E. (1978). *The market for human blood.* Lexington, MA: Lexington Books.

Howe, R. A. W. (1995). Redefining the transracial adoption controversy. *Duke Journal of Gender, Law and Policy, 2,* 131–164.

Howe, R. A. W. (1997). Transracial adoption (TRA): Old prejudices and discrimination float under a new halo. *The Boston University Public Interest Law Journal, 6*(2), 409–472.

Human Fertilisation and Embryology Authority. (1998). *Code of Practice*. London: Human Fertilisation and Embryology Authority.

Humphrey, M. (1986). Infertility as a marital crisis. *Stress Management, 2*, 221–224.

Humphrey, M. & Humphrey, H. (1988). *Families with a difference: Varieties of surrogate parenthood*. New York: Routledge.

Institute for Science, Law and Technology. (1998). *Biomedicine: ART into science: Regulation of fertility techniques*. Chicago: Illinois Institute of Technology, American Association for the Advancement of Science.

In re Adoption of Doe. (1994). 638 N.E.2d 181 Illinois. Sub nom In re. Petition of Kirchner. (1995). 649 N.E.2d 324 (Illinois).

Jacoby, N. (1999, April 5). Financing an adoption. CNN: The financial network. [On-line]. Available: http://cnnfn.com/1999/04/05/life/ q_adoption/[2000, Feb. 16].

Johnson v. Calvert. (1993). 5 Cal.4th 84, 851 P.2d 776.

Kingsberg, S. A., Applegarth, L. D., & Janata, J. W. (2000). Embryo donation programs and policies in North America: Survey results and implications for health and mental health professionals. *Fertility and Sterility, 73*(2), 215–220.

Kirk, H. D. (1964). *Shared fate*. New York: Free Press.

Kirk, H. D. (1985). *Adoptive kinship: A modern institution in need of reform*. Toronto: Butterworths.

Klock, S. C., Jacob M. C., & Maier, D. (1994). A prospective study of donor insemination recipients: Secrecy, privacy, and disclosure. *Fertility and Sterility, 62*, 477–484.

Klock, S., & Maier, D. (1991) Psychological factors related to donor insemination. *Fertility and Sterility, 56*, 489–495.

Kolata, G. (1997, November 23). Clinics selling embryos made for "adoption." *The New York Times*, p. A1, A34.

Kuhns, J. (1994). The sealed adoption records controversy: Breaking down the walls of secrecy. *Golden Gate University Law Review, 24*(1), 259–297.

Lamport, A. (1988). The genetics of secrecy in adoption, artificial insemination, and in vitro fertilization. *American Journal of Law and Medicine, 14*(1), 109–124.

Landau, R. (1999). Planned orphanhood. *Social Science & Medicine,* *49*(2), 185–196.

Lehr v. Robinson. (1983). 463 U.S. 248.

Lieberman, E. J. (1998). Adoption and identity. *Adoption Quarterly, 2*(2), 1–5.

Lifton, B. J. (1994). *Journey of the adopted self: A quest for wholeness.* New York: Basic Books.

Lightman, E. & Schlesinger, B. (1982). Pregnant adolescents in maternity homes: Some professional concerns. In R. R. Stuart & C. F. Wells (Eds.), *Pregnancy in adolescence: Needs, problems, and management* (pp. 363–406). New York: Van Nostrand Reinhold Company.

Lyke, M. L. (1999a). Costs for egg donations soar as demand rises and altruism wanes. *Seattle Post-Intelligencer.* Available: http://www.seattlep-i.com:80/lifestyle/egg31.shtml [1999, Sept. 1].

Lyke, M. L. (1999b). Egg donation—you wouldn't want to make it a career. *Seattle Post-Intelligencer.* Available: http://www.seattlep-i.com:80/lifestyle/risk31.shtml [1999, Sept. 1].

Macklin, R. (1991). Artificial means of reproduction and our understanding of the family. *Hastings Center Report*, January/February, 5–11.

Macklin, R. (1995). Artificial means of reproduction and our understanding of the family. In J. Howell & F. Sale (Eds.), *Life choices: A Hastings Center introduction to bioethics* (pp. 287–301). Washington, D.C.: Georgetown University Press.

Macklin, R. (1996). What is wrong with commodification? In C. Cohen (Ed.), *New ways of making babies: A case of egg donation* (pp. 106–120). Bloomington: Indiana University Press.

Macklin, R. & White, G. B. (1997). Assisted reproductive technologies, ads, and ethics: Philosophical, ethical, and clinical perspectives on the use of advertising in reproductive medicine. *Women's Health Issues, 7*(3), 127–131.

Mahlstedt, P. P. & Probasco, K. A. (1991). Sperm donors: Their attitudes toward providing medical and psychological information for recipient couples and donor offspring. *Fertility & Sterility, 56*(4,) 747–753.

Mahoney, J. (1995). Adoption as a feminist alternative to reproductive technology. In J. C. Callahan (Ed.), *Reproduction, ethics, and the law* (pp. 35–54). Bloomington: Indiana University Press.

Mahowald, M. B. (1996). Conceptual and ethical considerations in medically assisted reproduction. In M. M. Seibel & S. L. Crockin (Eds.), *Family building through egg and sperm donation: Medical, legal and ethical issues.* New York: Jones & Bartlett Publishers.

Mandell, B. R. (1973). *What are the children? A class analysis of foster care and adoption.* Lexington, MA: Lexington Books.

Mansnerus, L. (1998, October 26). Market puts price tags on the priceless. *The New York Times*, p. A1.

Mason, M. M. (1995). *Out of the shadows: Birthfathers' stories.* Edina, MN: O. J. Howard Publishing.

McHutchinson, J. (1986). *Relinquishing a child: The circumstances and effects of loss.* Unpublished paper. On file at the University of New South Wales, Australia.

McTaggart, L. (1980). *The baby brokers.* New York: Dial Press.

M.L.B. v. S.L.J. (1996). 519 U.S. 102.

Mead, R. (1999, August 9). Annals of reproduction: Eggs for sale. *The New Yorker*, pp. 56–65.

Melina, L. (1986). *Raising adopted children.* New York: Harper Perennial.

Meyer v. Nebraska. (1923). 262 U.S. 390.

Miall, C. (1987). The stigma of adoptive parent status: Perceptions of community attitudes toward adoption and the experience of informal social sanctioning. *Family Relations, 36*(1), 34–39.

Modell, J. S. (1994). *Kinship with strangers: Adoption and interpretations of kinship in American culture.* Berkeley: University of California Press.

Morrison, B. (2000, March 19). Lost and found. *The Independent (London)*, pp. 1, 11, 13, 14.

Neumann, P. J., Gharib, S. D., & Weinstein, M. C. (1994). The cost of a successful delivery with in vitro fertilization. *New England Journal of Medicine, 331*(4), 239–244.

The New York State Task Force on Life and the Law. (1998). *Assisted reproductive technologies: Analysis and recommendations for public policy.* New York: The New York State Task Force on Life and the Law.

Paulson, J. O., Haarmann, B. S., Salerno, R. L., & Asmar, P. (1988). An investigation of the relationship between emotional maladjustment and infertility. *Fertility and Sterility, 49*(2), 258–262.

Perry, T. L. (1998). Transracial and international adoption: Mothers, hierarchy, race and feminist legal theory. *Yale Journal of Law and Feminism, 10,* 101–164.

Pertman, A. (1998, March 9). Vying to be among the chosen. *The Boston Globe,* pp. A1, A10–A11.

Planned Parenthood v. Casey. (1992). 505 U.S. 833.

Prager, D. (1999). Men and adoption: Do you love your child or your seed? In C. Marshner & W. L. Pierce (Eds.), *Adoption factbook III* (pp. 362–364). Washington, DC: National Council for Adoption.

Ragoné, H. (1996). Chasing the blood tie: Surrogate mothers, adoptive mothers and fathers. *American Ethnologist, 23*(2), 352–365.

Reitz, M. & Watson, K. W. (1992). *Adoption and the family system.* New York: Guilford Press.

Richardson, V. (1999, Sept. 8). Adoption agency seeks parents for frozen embryos. *The Washington Times,* p. 8.

Robertson, J. A. (1988-89). Technology and motherhood: Legal and ethical issues in human egg donation. *Case Western Reserve Law Review, 39,* 1–38.

Romanchik, B. (1997, Summer). Birthparent transformation: Defining our public and self images. *Open Adoption: Birthparent, 13,* 1–2.

Rosenberg, E. B. (1992). *The adoption life cycle: The children and their families through the years.* New York: Free Press.

Rowland, R. (1985). The social and psychological consequences of secrecy in artificial insemination by donor (AID) programmes. *Social Science and Medicine, 21*(4), 391–396.

Rubin, R. (1998, December 8). One couple's surplus can fill void of another. *USA Today,* A1, A2.

Rubin, S. (1983). Letter to the Editor, School Paper, California State University. Northbridge, CA.

Rycus, J. S., Hughes, R. C., & Goodman, D. A. (1998). Adoption. In J. S. Rycus & R. C. Hughes (Eds.), *Field guide to child welfare* (Vol. 4) (p. 881–1038). Washington, DC: CWLA Press.

Sandelowski, M. (1995). A theory of the transition to parenthood of infertile couples. *Research in Nursing & Health, 18*(2), 123–132.

Sauer, M. V. (1996). Oocyte donation: Reflections on past work and future directions. *Human Reproduction, 11*(6), 1149–1155.

Saunders, B. (1996 Spring). Birthfathers come of age. *Birthparent, 8*, 1.

Schechter, M. & Bertocci, D. (1990). The meaning of search. In D. Brodzinsky & M. D. Schechter (Eds.), *The psychology of adoption* (pp. 62–92). New York: Oxford University Press.

Seibel, M. M., Kiessling, A. A., Bernstin, J., & Levia, S. R. (1993). *Technology and infertility: Clinical, psychosocial, legal, and ethical aspects*. New York: Springer-Verlag.

Shapiro, C. H. (1982). The impact of infertility on the marital relationship. *Social Casework, 63*(9), 387–393.

Shapiro, C. H. (1993). *When part of the self is lost: Helping clients heal after sexual and reproductive losses*. San Francisco: Jossey-Bass.

Smith, G. P. (1990). The case of Baby M: Love's labor lost. In L. Gostin (Ed.), *Surrogate motherhood: Politics and privacy* (pp. 233–242). Bloomington: Indiana University Press.

Sokoloff, B. Z. (1987). Alternative methods of reproduction: Effects on the child. *Clinical Pediatrics, 26*(1), 11–17.

Sorosky, A. D., Baran, A., & Pannor, R. (1984). *The adoption triangle*. Garden City, NY: Anchor Books.

South Australian Council on Reproductive Technology. (2000). *Conception by donation: Access to identifying information in the use of donated sperm, eggs and embryos in reproductive technology in South Australia*. Rundle Mall, South Australia: South Australian Council on Reproductive Technology.

Stephen, G. H. & Chandra, A. (2000). Use of infertility services in the United States: 1995. *Family Planning Perspectives, 32*(3), 132–137.

Trevison, C. (1997, October 7). Dispute over adoption records to continue. *The Tennessean*, p. 3B.

Triseliotis, J. (1973). *In search of origins: The experience of adopted people*. London: Routledge & Kegan Paul.

USA Today. (1999, September 16). Classified advertisements, p. 10D.

U.S. Department of Health and Human Services. (1996). *Assisted reproductive technology success rates: National summary and fertility clinic reports*. Washington, DC: Author.

Van Keppel, M. & Winkler, R. (1983, April 23). *The adjustment of relinquishing mothers in adoption: The results of a national study*. Presented at the first conference of the National Council for the

Single Woman and Her Child and the Association Representing Mothers Separated from their Children by Adoption, Adelaide, South Australia.

Verhovek, S. H. (2000, April 5). Debate on adoptees' rights stirs Oregon. *The New York Times*, p. A1, A20.

Vermont Statutes. (1999). Title 15A: Adoption Act. [On-line]. Available: http://www.leg.state.vt.us/statutes/title15a/chap007.htm#07-00103 [2000, June 8].

Vorzimer, A. W. (1998, January 20). Revisiting Jaycee B.: A different perspective. The American Surrogacy Center [On-line]. Available: http://www.surrogacy.com/legals/jaycee/jayceediff.html [2000, Mar. 10].

Ward, A. (1988, May 11). Written testimony, presented orally, at a public hearing on surrogacy conducted by the New Jersey Bioethics Commission, Newark, NJ.

Ward, M. (1998). The impact of adoption on the new parents' marriage. *Adoption Quarterly, 2*(2), 57–78.

Watson, K. W. (1999). Who cares if people are exploited by adoption? *Decree, 1*, 7–8.

Wells, S. (1993). Post-traumatic stress disorder in birth mothers. *Adoption & Fostering, 17*(4), 22–26.

Williams, L. S. (1992). Adoption actions and attitudes of couples seeking in vitro fertilization. *Journal of Family Issues, 13*(1), 99–113.

Winter, C. (1997, December 16). The biological imperative (Part 2 of The Fertility Race). MSNBC. Available: http://www.msnbc.com/news/130623.asp [1999, Nov. 11].

Wisconsin v. Yoder. (1972). 406 U.S. 205.

Wright, J., Bissonnette, F., Duchesne, C., Benoit, J., Sabovrin, S., & Girard, Y. (1991). Psychological distress and infertility: Men and women respond differently. *Fertility and Sterility, 55*(1), 100–108.

Zelizer, V. (1985). *Pricing the priceless child.* Princeton, NJ: Princeton University Press.

About the Author

Madelyn Freundlich is policy director for Children's Rights, Inc., New York, NY. She formerly served as the executive director of the Evan B. Donaldson Adoption Institute and as general counsel for the Child Welfare League of America. She is a social worker and lawyer whose work has focused on child welfare policy and practice for the past decade. She has authored a number of books and articles on child welfare law and policy. Her most recent writing has focused on the impact of welfare reform on foster care and special needs adoption; the role of race and culture in adoption; interstate adoption law and practice; genetic testing in adoption evaluations; and confidentiality in child welfare practice. Ms. Freundlich holds masters degrees in social work and public health and holds a JD and LLM.